GREAT FOOD,
Great Sex

GREAT FOOD,

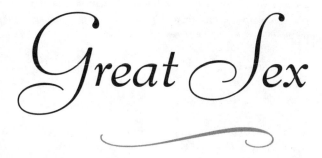

Great Sex

THE THREE FOOD FACTORS

FOR SEXUAL FITNESS

Robert Fried, Ph.D.,
and Lynn Edlen-Nezin, Ph.D.

BALLANTINE BOOKS

NEW YORK

Published in the United States by Ballantine Books, an imprint of The Random House Publishing Group, a division of Random House, Inc., New York.

BALLANTINE and colophon are registered trademarks of Random House, Inc.

Library of Congress Cataloging-in-Publication Data

Fried, Robert L.
    Great food, great sex: the three food factors for sexual fitness / Robert Fried and Lynn Edlen-Nezin.
        p.   cm.
    Includes bibliographical references and index.
    ISBN 0-345-48398-7
        1. Sex. 2. Diet. 3. Nutrition. 4. Physical fitness. 5. Sexual disorders—Diet therapy. 6. Sex (Biology)—Nutritional aspects. I. Edlen-Nezin, Lynn. II. Title.

RA788.F75 2006
616.6'90654—dc22   2005058511

Printed in the United States of America on acid-free paper

www.ballantinebooks.com

9 8 7 6 5 4 3 2 1

First Edition

Book design by Cassandra J. Pappas.

Is it not strange that desire should so many years outlive performance?

—WILLIAM SHAKESPEARE

Foreword

At a time when sexual dysfunction is on the rise, there has been a plethora of books recommending everything from exotic clothing, tantric yoga, and masterful oral sex to nutritional supplements and of course pharmaceutical products. So what do the brussels sprouts, nuts, and dark chocolate touted in this book have to do with great sex? Are they the new aphrodisiacs?

The real news is that great sex is not achieved through aphrodisiacs, but rather through good nutrition. *Great Food, Great Sex* proposes that the same diet that clogs the vessels of your heart can ultimately impair the blood flow to your sexual organs. This thesis is based on conclusive research evidence that up to 90 percent of reported sexual dysfunction in both men and women is *not* due to an emotional block but to an actual medical disorder largely related to diet. The authors' simple but elegant solution is to change your plate, not your mate; to concentrate your efforts in the produce department and the kitchen in order to reap rewards in the bedroom.

Great Food, Great Sex optimizes sexual health by outlining a nutritional method for (1) supplying the body with adequate nitric oxide—the essential fuel required for erection in men and engorgement and lubrication in women—and (2) ensuring the health of the endothelial tissues that line our arterial blood vessels with an optimal supply of antioxidants.

The American diet of highly processed, low-fiber foods that are high in refined carbohydrates and saturated fats is the enemy of good cardiovascular health as well as sexual vitality. As the authors point out, by the time the average American is forty-five years old, blood vessel walls may contain nearly half the atherosclerotic plaque that will accumulate in an expected lifetime. It is this plaque that interferes directly with sexual vitality by impeding adequate blood flow; thus the problem is not aging per se, but the lack in our daily diet of the nutrients that are necessary to protect the lining of our arterial blood vessels over the life span.

To make matters worse, the drugs that are often prescribed to help with cardiovascular conditions may further interfere with arousal and sexual functioning. And Viagra and similar drugs, appropriately credited with helping millions of men to regain sexual function, are still less than magic pills, and are not without risk for men with certain cardiovascular conditions. Importantly, for couples in whom only one partner is treated with drugs that promote erections, sex can become a scenario of vigorous penile thrusting, leaving a large percentage of women sexually unfulfilled and, in many cases, physically uncomfortable.

It is only in the past couple of decades that the clitoris has been clearly identified as women's primary sex organ, so sexual intercourse is only part of a woman's sexual function. Clinical trials with erectile dysfunction drugs have failed to show enhancement of low libido in women or help them become more orgasmic. To the contrary, *Great Food, Great Sex* is a nutritional program for men *and* women, providing benefits to both sexes by virtue of improved circulation.

Packed with voluminous information on the role of diet in sexual health, this book is a fascinating and witty read. It is worth buying for its well-researched information on nutrition alone; it is one of the most outstanding books I have ever seen on the subject.

Great Food, Great Sex is replete with solid information and fascinating details, such as the amount of antioxidants in leading brands of red and white wines. In addition, it includes specific eating plans and simple-to-prepare recipes for maintaining overall physical health, both above and below the belt.

Healthy food can be great food, and sex enjoyed by both partners is my definition of great sex. As a sex therapist with more than thirty years of experience (and author of the popular book *What to Do When* He *Has a Headache*), I find this plan an invaluable aid for clients—whose mental and physical zest I have long observed to be closely related to good nutrition. I encourage readers to plan a romantic trip to the grocery store, followed by the foreplay of a delicious meal. The rest I leave to your imagination.

—JANET L. WOLFE, Ph.D.
October 2005

Preface

In 1990, I was diagnosed with severe tachycardia and hypertension, a common feature in my family. My physician prudently prescribed medications to slow my heartbeat and to lower my blood pressure, and I soon began to know the meaning of "adverse side effects." I am not opposed to prescription medications—on the contrary, they save countless lives every day. But in those days, these medications interfered with my love life. Well, that certainly would not do! I was, after all, only fifty-five years old.

Molded into a traditional academic-scientist by many decades of university culture, I set about finding a science-based treatment for my cardiovascular conditions in the vast online universe of medical research publications (MEDLINE: Entrez PubMed). It is amazing what one can find there: As luck would have it, a smattering of scientists in various parts of the world were agonizing over the identity of a mysterious molecule that seemed to exert control over the way blood flows through our blood vessels. Cardiovascular scientists were tantalized by a hint that we were on the verge of a major breakthrough in cardiovascular physiology.

Two classes of neurotransmitters, *adrenergic* and *cholinergic* chemical messengers, control cardiovascular and heart function. Now, the scientists knew that this mysterious molecule was neither *adrenergic* nor *cholinergic* but a yet unknown third type, so they termed it NANC for non-adrenergic, non-cholinergic. Although the discovery of NANC was to earn three

American scientists the Nobel Prize in Medicine in 1998, it was a British scientist, Dr. Salvador Moncada, who unmasked it with the unlikely revelation that it is a gas, nitric oxide (NO).

NO causes constricted blood vessels to relax, thus lowering blood pressure. But where could I get some NO to lower mine? I thought of moving to Los Angeles, where smog holds a plentiful supply. But the answer was clearly to do it the way the body does it: It gets NO from the amino acid L-arginine. Could it be that something in my body was hampering NO production, thus raising my blood pressure? As it turns out, scientists soon discovered that this was precisely the problem in most hypertensives.

Amino acid L-arginine supplements can be found in plentiful supply in any health food store because body builders have been using it for years to help excrete dangerous excess ammonia built up due to strenuous muscle exercise. Experimenting with it and monitoring my blood pressure every day, I soon discovered that for me, 2,500 mg/day restored my blood pressure to normal levels.

But the bonus (pardon the pun) that I did not expect from this regimen is that **it significantly strengthened and prolonged erectile function.** Now I was on to something more to my liking. What quickly followed was the revelation that Pfizer, working with its own molecule (type 5 PDE inhibitor) that prolonged the effects in the body of L-arginine–derived NO as a blood pressure–lowering medication, discovered the same phenomenon, and that gave birth to Viagra.

I was so happy about all this that I decided to share my discovery of these discoveries—then still under wraps for the most part—with the consumer public. I teamed up with a brilliant colleague, the Manhattan-based physician Dr. Woodson C. Merrell, with whom I wrote *The Arginine Solution* (Warner Books, 1999). Dr. "Woody" is the most supportive medical colleague that I know when it comes to complementary/alternative medicine (CAM).

Medicine quickly caught on to the fact that NO lowers blood pressure, promotes heart function, lowers serum LDL (bad) cholesterol, and strengthens sexual function and vitality. Then early in 2004, I happened on clinical trials conducted by the National Heart, Lung, and Blood Institute (NHLBI) of the National Institutes of Health (NIH) to test a nutrition plan intended to raise NO for the treatment of cardiovascular and heart disease. Our government finally caught on that increasing NO is the way to go.

The NHLBI devised a nutrition plan consisting of recipes with foods that are rich NO-donors, as it were. These are the "greens and beans" (vegetables) rich in nitrogen compounds that deliver NO, and the "staminators" (meats, nuts, legumes) rich in L-arginine that deliver ample NO. With their permission, we reprint many of their recipes here.

Lots of NO means lots of Yes, and I thought you might want to know that. So, I teamed up with my nutrition-savvy colleague, Dr. Lynn Edlen-Nezin to shape all this into a workable NO-rich foods plan intended to help you promote a lifetime of cardiovascular and heart health accompanied by renewed sexual vitality and satisfying sexual performance.

—ROBERT FRIED

I first met Dr. Robert Fried as my professor of Learning Theory at Hunter College, and became enchanted with his dynamic lecture style, which included an impressive dramatic interpretation of the mating dance of the peacock. Little did I know that more than a quarter century later we would team up to help improve the mating dance of the human. I became Dr. Fried's teaching assistant and he helped me survive a bachelor degree in psychology with a minimum of psychic trauma.

At the time I decided to pursue a doctorate in health psychology. I had an established career as a certified personal trainer and fitness instructor, with a star-studded clientele. I spent as much time dispensing nutritional guidance as I did teaching my students to execute abdominal exercises. When I was accepted at The Einstein College of Medicine I continued to work with issues of nutrition and lifestyle modification with Dr. Judith Wylie-Rosett, a professor of clinical nutrition, and Dr. Charles Swencionis, a health psychologist, in a number of National Heart, Lung, and Blood Institute–funded research projects on weight loss, hypertension, and hypercholesterolemia reduction. I was continually impressed with how poorly knowledge correlated with behavior, and I continued to believe that there had to be a more powerful incentive to modify nutritional and dietary behavior.

A number of years passed, during which I continued to work in research on women's health and nutrition, and then nutrition and cancer prevention. I changed careers and moved into advertising and marketing of health care. I had essentially lost touch with Dr. Fried until he walked through the door of a Chinese restaurant where I was having dinner with my family. We have that rare and wonderful kind of relationship in which both parties can resume contact as if they had seen each other the day before, instead of years ago. We shared stories of our experiences over the past years, and discovered that we had both moved into nutrition and behavior as core interests and professional pursuits. He told me of his idea to continue his exploration of L-arginine and sexuality by concentrating on diet, and our book idea was born.

I am so excited by our approach to modifying dietary behavior through sexual function because I sincerely believe it is intrinsically more appealing to most of us than the continued obsessive focus on waistlines. Despite all the public awareness of the health risks of our typical national diet, our population grows fatter and more sedentary by the year, so the health messaging is clearly ineffective. We hope that by turning our readers on to the nutrition-sex connection, they will be able to turn on their sex lives, turn up their metabolism, and permanently restructure their eating habits for a healthier and happier life.

Dr. Fried's rigorous academic approach to research mirrors my standards (learned as his student) and makes me confident that our program will not be added to the growing list of unsubstantiated fad diets.

We hope you enjoy the program as much as we enjoyed creating it.

—LYNN EDLEN-NEZIN

Acknowledgments

We owe a profound debt of gratitude to our literary agent, Alice F. Martell, without whose unwavering support and helpful suggestions this book project would have remained an intellectual discussion.

We also wish to express our appreciation to Mary Bahr, for her humor, understanding, and consummate attention to detail and organization that helped our book take shape. To Caroline Sutton, senior editor, Random House, we award a bushel of chocolate-covered strawberries for her patience and faith in this project.

Special thanks are also due Stuart Nezin for help with the illustrations in our book, and to Casey and Stuart both for their gracious tolerance of the long hours their mother and wife spent working with Bob to make this book a reality.

Our thanks to Dr. Andrei Voustianiouk for his tireless efforts in helping to assemble our extensive bibliography. We wish also to thank the following sources—journals and publishers—for permission to quote text or reproduce tables and figures:

- Elsevier.
- Lawrence Erlbaum Associates, Inc.
- Lippincott Williams & Wilkins Co.
- *Mayo Clinic Proceedings*.

- Springer-Verlag GmbH.
- The American Society for Nutritional Sciences.
- The Cleveland Clinic Foundation.
- United States Department of Agriculture (USDA) Nutrient Data Laboratory.

Contents

Introduction

Love never dies a natural death. It dies because we don't know how to replenish its source.

—ANAÏS NIN

Welcome to a new age of sexual fitness. Regardless of where you are on the sexual continuum, *Great Food, Great Sex* can enhance your sex life and that of your partner. You may already enjoy a satisfying sex life but would welcome improvement, or, like a surprising number of Americans of all ages, your personal sexual activity may be minimal. While there are many possible reasons for loss of sexual vigor, we now know that *most sexual dysfunction has a medical explanation*—and, fortunately, a physiological solution.

Great Food, Great Sex outlines an eating plan that will supercharge your sex life. Based on recent scientific discoveries—the very same information that led to the creation of Viagra and other pharmaceutical sex drugs—we show you how to get a safe, natural "dose" of what your body needs to function at its sexual peak using everyday foods. *Great Food, Great Sex* doesn't promise to make you a better lover, but on this plan you will be a healthier lover. Without relying on aphrodisiacs, or any particular sexual technique, our program can increase the stamina and sexual enjoyment of both men and women, young and old, and people at every level of sexual activity.

Our program works because it separates myth from fact. And the facts suggest that if you want to see an improvement in your sex life, you are not alone.

WHAT'S WRONG WITH THIS PICTURE?

Advertising is out of sync with reality. Despite the ubiquitous display of young, beautiful bodies in every magazine and major motion picture, despite the mainstreaming of nudity and sexually explicit scenes on prime-time television, in bedroom after bedroom across the country the thrill is gone. Our media culture is oversexualized, but most of us are undersexed.

According to current estimates, about 30 percent of adult men and 40 percent of adult women are at risk for some degree of sexual dysfunction. This means that approximately seventy million men and women out of a population of two hundred million Americans do not have fully functional sex lives.

Americans have significantly less impressive sex lives than the media seem to suggest. In an ABC News *Primetime Live* survey of 1,501 American adults conducted by telephone on August 2 through 9, 2004, overall only 7 percent of the US adult population reports having sex four or more times per week, while 18 percent report having no sex at all.

Among couples who've been together less than three years, 42 percent do not describe their sex lives as "very exciting." After more than ten years, that number jumps to 72 percent. And sex occurs several times a week for 72 percent of new couples but only 32 percent of long-term couples.

Perhaps it is not surprising that a culture so frustrated and disappointed in the bedroom would be obsessed—if popular culture is any indication—with sex. And with good reason: Apart from the obvious human desire to enjoy lovemaking, there are other benefits to having a healthy and fulfilled sex life.

An emerging and intriguing branch of economics called the economics of happiness seeks to identify and quantify the factors or activities that determine happiness. Social scientists have determined that sex and money are related in a very interesting way.

Most authorities on well-being recognize two key factors, sex and money, as having the most effect on the four primary categories that together form the way we judge the overall quality of our life: circumstances, aspirations, comparison with others, and disposition or outlook on life.

Recent data from the General Social Surveys (GSS) of the United States estimate that 12 percent of Americans describe their lives as not too happy, 58 percent say they are pretty happy, and 30 percent say they are very happy (GSS Question 157, 1988–2000).

How important is sex? According to analysis of the GSS data, sexual activity enters strongly into the happiness equation. The more sex a person has, the happier that person feels, and dividing the data into age groups does not change the correlation. Both men and women derive happiness from sex, and those who report having the most frequent sex report the greatest happiness.

A survey of one thousand employed women revealed that sex is rated as the activity that yields the single largest amount of happiness, while commuting to and from work yields the lowest levels (Kahneman, Krueger, et al., 2003). According to the ABC News *Primetime Live* poll American Sex Survey (October 21, 2004), having an exciting sex life contributes to a happy marriage, and a happy marriage contributes to life satisfaction. But according to the GSS, 40 percent of American females over the age of forty and 20 percent of men in the same age group did not have sexual intercourse over the past year.

In an interview with *The New York Times,* Drs. Blanchflower and Oswald, the authors of a joint US and British research publication on the economics of happiness, discussed a mathematical model called econometrics by which they made the following calculations:

- Great sex at least once a week is worth about $50,000 in happiness. This means that having great sex at least once a week will make the average American adult as happy as having $50,000 in the bank.

- The emotional uplift of a long-lasting marriage is worth $100,000 in the bank, while a divorce causes about a $66,000 debit in happiness.

What about money? The GSS concludes that although greater wealth is associated with greater happiness, the wealthy are not having more sex.

Finally, contrary to popular myth, more is not necessarily merrier: A person needs only one sexual partner to be sexually fulfilled.

SEX—FOR THE HEALTH OF IT

In addition to contributing to a sense of general well-being, whether you are a man or a woman, frequent satisfying sex contributes significantly to health. Dr. Deepak Chopra writes that having sex three times a week for a year is the caloric equivalent of running 75 miles (sexualhealth.com). Sexual intercourse burns approximately 150 calories per hour.

Beneficial hormones are stimulated in both men and women during and after sex, blood flow to the brain and other organs is increased, and the experience of orgasm helps many people reduce stress. Sex acts as an analgesic and can help relieve aches and pains. The best we can say for abstinence is that it's best to practice it in moderation. Still, despite an obvious upside, an impressive number of us do not seem to be having very satisfying sex lives, and people are looking for answers.

The Drug Solution

Our new, medically accurate physiological understanding of sexual dysfunction dates from a revolutionary breakthrough based on the work of three American researchers, Drs. R. F. Furchgott, L. J. Ignarro, and F. Murad, who shared the 1998 Nobel Prize in Medicine. They determined that insufficient production of nitric oxide (NO), a gas heretofore not known to have any biological action in our body, results in inadequate blood flow. Inadequate blood flow to the sex organs was later identified as the primary cause of male impotence. This discovery ultimately led to the development of Viagra, which works by prolonging the activity of NO in the body.

Viagra and other drugs that treat erectile dysfunction by utilizing NO technology have essentially banished Freud from the bedroom. This new physiological knowledge has helped to *medicalize* sexual dysfunction, resulting in better diagnosis and treatment without the stigmas long associated with the loss of sexual vitality.

With the wide availability of prescription medications, record numbers of men have talked to their health care practitioners about erectile dysfunction. Our national preoccupation with aging has helped contribute to the phenomenal success of these sex drugs. Thanks to medications such as Viagra, Levitra, and Cialis, many men now feel they have a shot at successful lovemaking despite weakened hearts, joints, and musculature. For many of us, sexuality equals youthfulness, and restoring sexual function is a way to turn back the clock.

It is important to emphasize that prescription sex drugs are not for all and should only be resorted to with the supervision of a physician. These medications can cause a precipitous drop in blood pressure in some people, putting them at serious risk. Finally, according to a recent report, only one in three men benefits from prescription sex drugs, and it is still unclear if and how these drugs help women.

Hope in Hormones

Hormone therapy is also used to treat sexual dysfunction, but seems to help only a small percentage of people. Interestingly, many men diagnosed with impotence have levels of testosterone well within the normal range. In fact, average testosterone levels in healthy men are about the same at age *seventy* as at age *twenty*—and hormone production actually peaks at about age forty-five (Wagner and Green, 1981).

Testosterone replacement in women, a treatment common for some time, often involves using testosterone patches developed for men. Testosterone products specifically formulated at appropriate dosages for women have now been developed.

Unlike the drugs for erectile dysfunction, testosterone replacement in women does seem to help improve libido. Unfortunately, although testosterone supplements help treat loss of libido, vaginal atrophy, and dryness, women taking these male hormones can experience undesirable symptoms of virilization such as growth of facial hair, a deeper voice, and acne.

STEP UP TO THE PLATE

We offer an alternative approach. You will learn how and why nutritional habits are the cause of many cases of sexual dysfunction and how easy it is to develop new nutritional habits that work to reverse the problem.

The eating plan that we offer in *Great Food, Great Sex* supports your body with the nutrition it needs for healthy sexual function. Designed to satisfy two essential drives—sex and hunger—this simple, easy-to-implement program integrates up-to-date scientific knowledge with a food plan that improves sexual function by addressing the body's complete sexual physiology.

Our eating plan promotes the healthy circulation needed for satisfying lovemaking in both men and women without relying on supplements, special foods, or radical eating modifications. The foods recommended in *Great Food, Great Sex* combine to guide you into a nutritional state of health and balance in which all tissues of the body, including the sex organs, are receiving the blood supply needed for optimal function.

Great Food, Great Sex can help put you on the road to a lifetime of satisfying sex, while also providing health benefits above and beyond sexual pleasure. We outline a basic six-week nutritional plan with principles that can be followed for a lifetime, and started at any age. Best of all, the ingredients you need for *Great Food, Great Sex* are as close to you as the nearest grocery store.

By mindfully selecting the particular foods that we eat every day, we can easily meet the physiological requirements for active and vital sexual function. With no more effort than you put into eating, you can tank up at mealtime with the high-octane sex fuels that nature provides for a delicious, exciting, and fun lifetime of sexual fulfillment. While *Great Food, Great Sex* does not rely on aphrodisiacs that might improve libido or allure, when sexual performance is enhanced it is both easier and more enjoyable to have sex more often. So enough foreplay; let's get down to business.

GREAT FOOD,
Great Sex

What's Under the Hood

Pushing Freud Out of Bed

The sexual needs of men and women may differ categorically, but there is considerable overlap, particularly with regard to function. And in terms of our understanding of sexual function, science has come a long way, baby.

Drs. Masters and Johnson were the first to bring sex science into the bedroom more than thirty years ago. They carefully mapped out and described the hydraulics and the mechanics of the "sexual act." Based on their daring and astonishing scientific observations, they showed how men and especially women go through distinct stages of sexual arousal before one can insert "tab A" into "slot A."

It took many years for the mechanics and physiology of sex to seep into psychiatry and sex therapy. Armed with theories about the Oedipus conflict and other assorted obscure neuroses, conventional psychological wisdom fought Masters and Johnson tooth and nail. Men, but more often women, were made to feel that their sexual problems were "all in their head." This bias kept many patients from ever admitting they were suffering from sexual dysfunction.

Even today, many of us have little to no knowledge of the basics of sex and sexuality. Despite the sexual revolution and easy access to information about all aspects of sex, a recent article in *Cosmopolitan* magazine (October 2003) featured instructions on how to "find your G-spot" (Rush, 2003). It seems that even among the well educated, savvy, and sophisticated, there is a dearth of important knowledge about sexual landmarks.

This a book about enhancing sexual vitality and performance by extracting the constituents that fuel it from three selected food categories. This is not a book about reproductive biology. However, as experts in the health and behavioral sciences, we are often astonished at how little many people know about their sex organs and how they work, and how often that ignorance impedes their sexual satisfaction as well as their emotional well-being.

The next section is a guide to the most relevant anatomical and physiological details of our sexual equipment. Knowing how our sexual organs work will also help you understand how and why the program offered in *Great Food, Great Sex* works. Here are the knowledge and the power to make you an expert in keeping the necessary plumbing in tip-top shape.

In the long run, satisfactory sexual performance depends mainly on maintaining proper cardiovascular function so that when you are sexually aroused, blood flow to the sex organs increases as needed to engorge the tissues of those organs. For men, this is experienced as an erection, while for women, it may be perceived as warmth and lubrication of the vaginal tissue. The biochemical sequence that translates amorous arousal into physical arousal creates a cascade that's similar in men and women, but by no means identical.

In addition to visible changes that occur during sex, complicated chemical activities go on in the body. An extremely basic explanation of the key steps in sexual arousal (omitting a number of intermediary enzymes that play a key role in this sequence but add little to our understanding of the sequence) is as follows:

The brain releases acetylcholine (ACh) as a result of sexual arousal. The bloodstream carries it to the blood vessels in the sex organs, where it signals the vessel lining, the endothelium, to release a gas, nitric oxide (NO). NO then causes the endothelium to release a vasodilator substance, cyclic guanosine monophosphate (cGMP). cGMP relaxes the blood vessels and causes increased blood flow to the sex organs for erection in men or engorgement in women.

$$ACh \rightarrow NO \rightarrow cGMP = physical\ arousal$$

After sex, the enzyme phosphodiesterase type 5 (PDE5) deactivates cGMP:

$$PDE5 \rightarrow cGMP + post\text{-}arousal$$

As you will see below, this is the sequence for penile erection in men; a very similar sequence is involved in lubrication and vaginal and clitoral engorgement in women. Engorgement is an obvious prerequisite for men in attaining an erection, but also directly contributes to pleasurable sensations in women.

THE ALL-IMPORTANT ENDOTHELIUM

Arterial blood vessels carry oxygenated blood from the lungs to body tissues. They range in size from large arteries down to smaller arterioles and finally to capillaries. Capillaries connected to the venules carry deoxygenated blood back to the lungs. Venules are the smallest of the veins in the body.

Arteries are made up of muscle rings and three major wall layers. Most important to us is the endothelium, the inner cell lining of the vessels. It is this cell lining that determines the way that the vessels control blood flow by their ability to expand or to constrict.

The endothelium responds to a number of the so-called action hormones (noradrenaline and others) that may constrict the vessels to increase blood pressure. But most important, the endothelium produces the gas nitric oxide (NO) to relax the blood vessels and increase blood flow to organs ranging from the heart to the sex organs.

The endothelium can be considered to be the business end of the blood vessels, and its control by NO is the discovery that resulted in the awarding of the 1998 Nobel Prize to three American scientists. No one knew before that event that the endothelium was anything but a sheet lining the inside of blood vessels. No one even knew that it served any biological purpose—much less that it actually controls the blood vessels. The endothelium is so critical to blood flow that capillaries are nothing but tubular structures made up entirely of endothelial cells.

As you'll read in detail throughout this book, the Great Food, Great Sex eating plan is built around three Food Factors that each supply the body with the ability to synthesize NO. Yet as powerful as these Food Factors are, they cannot compensate for inadequate hormone levels. Conversely, hormone levels may be adequate and sexual dysfunction may still occur if there is inadequate NO for this reason:

Sexual function requires an adequate arterial blood supply to the endothelium. If the neurochemical message does not reach the target, or the endothelium is too damaged to respond, the sequence is in vain. Damaged endothelial tissue results in impaired blood flow to the genitals during sexual arousal.

Our typical American diet is particularly damaging to the endothelium, and this impaired blood flow is the principal culprit in sexual dysfunction in men, and also in women up to menopause (Bernardo, 2001; Park, Goldstein, et al., 1997).

Medical science has made enormous strides in finally unraveling the mechanism of sexual arousal and response and also what damages it. One of the principal culprits is elevated serum low-density lipoprotein (LDL) (bad) cholesterol and its frequent result, atherosclerosis (hardening of the arteries).

Scientists from the University of South Carolina have found that impotence is a very compelling reason to avoid bad cholesterol: Men with lower blood levels of the bad LDL cholesterol or higher levels of the good high-density lipoprotein (HDL) cholesterol are less likely to develop erectile dysfunction (ED) (Nikoobakht, Nasseh, and Pourkasmaee, 2005). In a similar study, men with total cholesterol levels over 240 mg/dl had nearly double the risk of ED, compared with men with readings around 180 or less. The researchers concluded that atherosclerosis impedes blood flow to the penis and thus constitutes a primary cause of impotence.

It is evident now that antioxidant-rich foods protect the body from the oxidation of LDL cholesterol. There is also overwhelming evidence that arginine can both lower serum levels of LDL cholesterol and even reverse the process of plaque deposition. The Great Food, Great Sex program supplies generous amounts of NO, antioxidants, and arginine—the three Food Factors the body needs for maximum sexual vitality.

THE OWNER'S GUIDE TO MALE SEXUAL ANATOMY AND FUNCTION

We are living in an era of impressive lifestyle-altering pharmaceutical breakthroughs in the treatment of impotence. To understand how and why these products work (the same principles upon which the Great Food, Great Sex program is based), it helps to know how an erection actually comes about.

The anatomy of the penis is somewhat complex. Think of the structure as three cylinders of sponge-like tissue. Two are corpus cavernosa; a third cylinder is the spongeosum. In order to have and maintain an erection, the cylinders need to fill with blood. Blood is pumped into the penis under

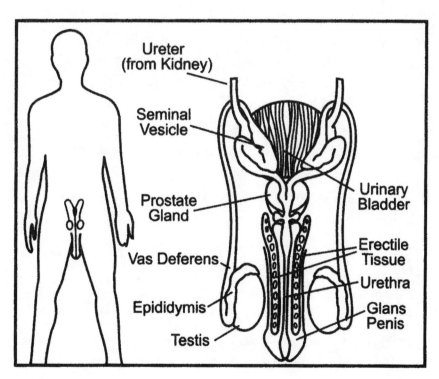

Figure 1.1: Male reproductive system. Reproduced with permission from Stuart Nezin, New York, NY, 2005.

body pressure. The expanding chambers compress the veins in the penis, slowing blood outflow.

The urethra is the inner tube that carries the urine and the ejaculate (a combination of semen and various other glandular fluids). The knobby head of the penis is called the glans. Blood flows to the penis by two very small arteries that come from the systemic aorta, the main artery that courses downward from the heart. These arteries are the same size as the arteries to your finger. If these blood vessels become blocked, blood cannot get to the penis. High-fat, low-vegetable, and low-fruit diets contribute directly to blocked vessels.

All three chambers of the penis are lined with endothelial tissue, as are arterial blood vessels. You might even think of these chambers as enlargeable blood vessels.

When you feel sexually turned on, the brain releases the neurotransmitter substance acetylcholine (ACh) into the bloodstream in the sex organs. Then:

- ACh then causes the endothelium in the blood vessels and in the spongy penis chambers to produce an enzyme called nitric oxide synthase (eNOS) that helps to produce the gas nitric oxide. This is derived most commonly from the amino acid arginine or, alternatively, from nitrogen compounds in foods.

- NO then triggers the release of yet another enzyme-induced neurotransmitter, cGMP.

- At the command of cGMP, the blood vessels relax, permitting increased blood inflow to the penis.

- As the chambers of the penis engorge, the sudden surge of blood into those chambers exerts pressure on the veins.

- Now inflow is greater than outflow, and the penis remains erect so long as there is a continuous production of cGMP mediated by NO.

- At the end of sexual activity, cGMP is disabled by the enzyme PDE5, and NO production decreases, causing the penis to return to its flaccid state.

The prostate gland surrounds a small section of the urethra between the urinary bladder and the penis. It secretes a lubricant fluid, which contributes about 15 to 30 percent of the volume of semen and enhances sperm motility. A set of small glands lying just below the prostate, on either side of the urethra, secretes a lubricant mucous substance that reduces the acidity of semen.

The scrotum, a pouch-like extension of the abdomen, is divided into two compartments, each containing a testicle where sperm originate. The production of sperm and their survival requires that they be maintained at a temperature about 3 degrees Fahrenheit below body temperature. When exposed to cold, a muscle called the cremaster elevates the testicles, bringing them closer to the body, thus warming them.

The enzyme PDE5 that deactivates cGMP production is a safety mechanism to limit the duration of an erection because, strictly speaking, an erection interferes with the normal flow of blood through the penis, increasing inflow at the expense of outflow. Viagra and the other drugs in its class are known as PDE5 inhibitors. These drugs work by blocking the safety valve and increasing the duration of the action of cGMP, thereby prolonging the erection.

Even though it has a very short life, once NO is released into the bloodstream it can cause blood vessels to relax throughout the body. (It has been noted that the concentration of NO released in the sex organs is greater than that released elsewhere in the body, leading to the theory that the sex organs have their own specific form of the enzyme eNOS.) This bodywide relaxation effect is why patients taking prescription heart medications that cause NO release, such as nitroglycerin or nitrate chest patches, are advised not to use drugs like Viagra. In these patients, release of cGMP can cause blood pressure to plummet to dangerously and sometimes irreversibly low levels, with potentially serious consequences.

THE OWNER'S GUIDE TO FEMALE SEXUAL ANATOMY AND FUNCTION

Although men may be from Mars and women from Venus, the same ACh-NO-cGMP sequence that operates in men operates in women as well. There are, however, some additional complexities that impact sexual function, relating to both the anatomy of a woman's sexual organs and her hormone status.

The female sensory sexual organs are much more complex than a man's, and they are largely internal. The sensory structures are also less

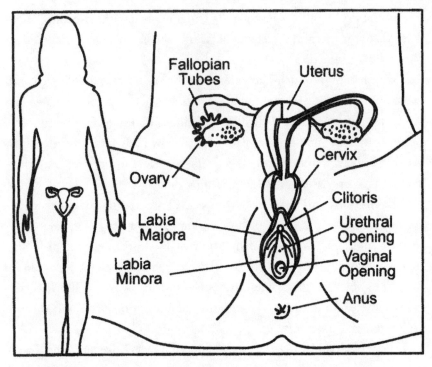

Figure 1.2: Female reproductive system. Reproduced with permission from Stuart Nezin, New York, NY, 2005.

clearly delineated from the surrounding vaginal tissue. In addition, a uniquely female sequence of arousal leads to orgasm in women.

More than a Vagina

The vulva includes the two sets of lips—the labia majora and labia minora—as well as the clitoris, the "urethral" opening (meatus), and the vaginal opening. The labia majora are fatty folds that fuse with the mons veneris or mound of Venus. The mound of Venus protects the pubic bone from the impact of sexual intercourse. The labia minora are smaller folds that become part of the vaginal mucosa, joining to form the prepuce, or fold of skin covering the tip of the clitoris. The clitoral prepuce is the female counterpart of the foreskin.

The Clitoris

The clitoris is a complex organ connecting nerves, tissues, muscles, and ligaments that react with one another when a woman is aroused. The clitoris shares structural similarities with the penis. This helps explain why understimulation of the clitoris may often result in an inability to experience orgasm.

The tip of the clitoris, or glans, is covered by a hood similar to the foreskin of the penis. The clitoris extends deep beneath the surface of the vulva and at the top, connects to the pubic bone; beneath the glans, splitting into a wishbone shape or crura (plural for *crus,* meaning "legs"), extending under the sides of the vagina down toward the anus. Medical science estimates that the sensitive glans contains up to eight thousand nerve endings, making that area extremely sensitive to stimulation.

The Vagina

The vagina is essentially a tube that connects the uterus with the chamber of the external genitals. It allows transport of sperm to the uterus and is also the passage for the birth of a newborn. It is made of a thick connective tissue layer containing blood vessels lined by epithelium cells that cover a dense layer of small blood vessels (capillaries). Three sets of skeletal muscles surround the vagina, including the pelvic floor muscles (pubococcygeus).

The G-Spot

The G-spot is an area of spongy erectile tissue in the vault of the vagina above the urethra, approximately 1 to 2 inches inside the vaginal opening on the front wall of the vagina. This erotic, sensitive area is located in closer relation to the bladder base than the urethra. The G-spot represents that part of the urethra that contains the periglandular or paraurethral tissue, corresponding to the female equivalent of the prostate. These glands are present to a greater or lesser degree in about 90 percent of women.

Lubrication

The surface cells of the epithelium undergo hormone-related changes during the menstrual cycle. The lubrication produced on a daily basis is usually not sufficient for intercourse without discomfort, so nature provides a mechanism to produce additional lubrication as part of the arousal process.

During sexual arousal, fluid appears within seconds at the entrance to the vagina in the form of bead-like droplets that have a smooth, slippery quality. These droplets merge to create a film that can partially decrease the acidity of the vaginal basal fluid. Contrary to common assumptions, there are no glands inside the vagina that increase vaginal lubrication on sexual arousal. Lubrication is supplied by glands external to the vagina. This is why many women find sex more comfortable with the addition of a lubricant before intercourse.

The Benefits of a Lube Job

Thumb through any popular magazine devoted to women and you will see a preponderance of advertisements for very expensive moisturizing products. Women today moisturize their hair, lips, eyes, and skin, often with a different product devoted to each body part. Given our preoccupation with aging, and our efforts to ward off dehydration, we might well ask why so many women neglect the moisture needs of their sexual organs.

The benefits of adequate lubrication, particularly in women who may be experiencing menopausal changes, cannot be overemphasized. Adequate lubrication can mean the difference between truly enjoyable sex and painful intercourse. Application of lubricants can become a pleasurable part of foreplay for many couples. A number of excellent products are on the market, ranging from the purely functional to the more playful.

Extensive medical research has shown conclusively that the blood flow changes that engorge the vagina and clitoris in sexual arousal are the same as those that engorge the penis in erection. The blood supply to the vagina is similarly under the control of the NO-cGMP sequence (Hoyle, Stones, et al., 1996). When a woman is "turned on," the blood supply to the vagina walls rapidly increases and at the same time the outflow of blood in the tissues is reduced, creating swelling (engorgement).

Medical researchers were surprised to discover the presence of nitric oxide synthase in human clitoral tissue, although this should have come as no surprise given the tissue and structural similarities to the penis. Because of the physiological similarities between men and women, researchers continue to suggest that PDE5 inhibitors such as Viagra, Cialis, and Levitra should be more extensively tested as treatment for female sexual dysfunction (FSD) (Gragasin, Michelakis, et al., 2004). Trials of Viagra in women have been inconclusive, however, for reasons detailed below.

A WORD ABOUT FEMALE SEXUAL DESIRE

In both men and women, it is important to draw a distinction between desire and performance. Currently available medications for sexual dysfunction, excepting hormone therapy, do not directly alter desire or libido.

As we learn more about sexual dysfunction, our models are changing. The original model, proposed by Masters and Johnson more than fifty years ago, is a simple progression from excitement to plateau and on to orgasm and resolution. A more holistic model, developed by Whipple and Brash-McGreer, tracks behavior from seduction through sensations, surrender, and reflection in an iterative pattern within which the Masters and Johnson phases can occur. This model is based on the understanding that many women do not move progressively and sequentially through the phases of the Masters and Johnson model and that behavior is modified by experience. This new model does not assume that sexual response in women is identical to that of men.

Sex educator and researcher Beverly Whipple, Ph.D., R.N., F.A.A.N., professor emeritus at Rutgers University, has proposed that the response in women is generally not linear. Sexual arousal may occur without desire, and as we have seen from the statistics, desire and arousal may not lead to orgasm.

This model underscores that it takes two to tango and that sex, especially for many women, is as much an emotional experience as a physical one—if not more so. Because Viagra and similar drugs only address the physical aspects of sex, they do not appear to significantly help women with low libido or HSDD (hypoactive sexual desire disorder).

Now that you know how it's supposed to work, let's talk about how and why it sometimes doesn't.

2

Sexual Dysfunction in Men and Women

It's Not in Your Head, It's in Your Heart

We are psychologists, and we have no wish to dismiss important psychological issues associated with sexuality in men and women. At the same time, however, we strongly believe that it is time to put physical and psychological issues into perspective. For both men and women, the vast majority of problems with sexual function are not psychological. Research has conclusively demonstrated that up to 90 percent of reported sexual dysfunction in both men and women is due not to an emotional block but to an actual medical disorder largely related to diet.

The following medical conditions, the majority of which are intimately related to dietary habits and practices, can directly impact and impair sexual function:

- Hypertension.
- Heart disease.
- Diabetes.
- Atherosclerosis.
- Obesity.

- Age-related hormone deficiency in women.

- Side effects of medications.

Medicine is becoming increasingly more knowledgeable about vascular (blood vessel) risk factors in impotence (Sullivan, Keoghane, et al., 2001). Diabetes is high on the list because it causes severe damage to the endothelium of the arterial blood vessels and to the heart.

A recent study in Finland determined that diabetes topped the list of risk factors for impotence, outpacing hypertension and heart disease (Shiri, Koskimaki, et al., 2003). Obesity seems to be especially threatening to sexual vitality—not because people who are overweight tend not to feel sexy, but because obesity is strongly associated with endothelial arterial blood vessel disease (Chung, Sohn, et al., 1999).

THE CARDIO—SEX CONNECTION

Current population health statistics tell us two startling facts about the adult American population: First, sexual dysfunction is epidemic, and second, cardiovascular and heart disease are epidemic. According to the Centers for Disease Control (CDC), more than 930,000 Americans die of cardiovascular disease (CVD) each year. That's one death every thirty-four seconds, day in and day out, most commonly among people sixty-five and older. But the incidence in those ages fifteen through thirty-four is increasing.

Almost one-quarter of our population—sixty-four million Americans—now lives with CVD: Coronary heart disease and stroke account for disability in more than one million of us each year. These statistics strongly resemble the equally widespread incidence of sexual dysfunction in Americans—seventy million.

The difference between these two statistics, six million, is most likely attributable to erectile dysfunction (ED) in men and female sexual dysfunction (FSD), which precede by just a few years diagnoses of cardiovascular disease—hypertension, atherosclerosis, heart disease, and stroke. In fact, ED and FSD are now said to warn us of impending cardiovascular disease.

A recent medical report titled "Is Erectile Dysfunction a Marker for Cardiovascular Disease?" concluded, "There is now significant evidence that erectile dysfunction (ED) can be a symptom of cardiovascular disease, and act as a marker for disease progression" (Kirby, Jackson, et al., 2001). The journal *Heart* has similarly noted that erectile dysfunction is a common condition, and that mounting evidence suggests it to be predominantly due to cardiovascular disease. "Cardiovascular risk factor control may be the key to preventing ED" (Solomon, Man, et al., 2003).

Not only is sexual dysfunction now thought to be a symptom of cardiovascular disease, but it may also predict CVD's severity. We show you in a later section that the parallel phenomenon in women is compounded by hormone depletion in menopause. To address the relationship between cardiovascular health and sexual dysfunction fully, we've got to dispense with a few myths and describe the fascinating mechanics of the sex act.

THE VASCULOGENIC THEORY OF SEXUAL DYSFUNCTION

One potential explanation proposed for sexual dysfunction in men is that a cardiovascular defect inhibits the endothelium of arterial blood vessels from responding to the NO-cGMP physical arousal sequence. Known as the vasculogenic theory of sexual dysfunction, this theory was originally thought not to apply to women, because women tend to complain more of loss of desire and orgasmic difficulties—problems related more to hormone imbalances or to emotional issues. Medicine now alerts us that cadiovascular diseases are equally likely to cause sexual arousal disorder in women as in men, citing diabetes and coronary heart disease as being the same risks to lovemaking for women as for men (Salonia, Munarris, & Montorsi, 2004).

Today researchers are realizing that many women may also be suffering from vasculogenic sexual dysfunction due to endothelial problems with the NO-cGMP sequence. In fact, before Viagra was marketed, an article coauthored by Dr. I. Goldstein, the developer of Viagra, concluded that atherosclerosis may be the culprit in insufficient vaginal and clitoral engorgement (Park, Goldstein, et al., 1997). For women diagnosed with vasculogenic sexual dysfunction, a product such as Viagra may be a viable treatment option.

As noted above, in 1997, investigators at the Johns Hopkins Hospital announced that they had isolated the nitric oxide synthase enzyme, eNOS, in the human clitoris. Their discovery indicates that the blood vessels of the clitoris respond to NO in the same way the penis does (Burnett, Calvin, et al., 1997). This understanding led the authors to conclude that the same arousal mechanisms may be operating in women as in men (D'Amati, di Gioia, et al., 2002). This has tremendous implications for the spectrum of sexual function in women. The Great Food, Great Sex program addresses vascular blood flow by providing a daily supply of nutrients to promote nitric oxide production.

In a 2001 study by the dynamic medical sister team, Drs. Berman and Berman, sildenafil (Viagra) was found to be effective and well tolerated by women with female sexual arousal disorder (FSAD—anorgasmicity) and postmenopausal women. Their study shows that when women take Viagra, blood flow increases to the vagina and lengthens, widens, and lubricates it during the arousal state. Blood flow also increases to the labia minora and clitoris, resulting in swelling and engorgement. One study went so far as to conclude that ". . . tissue organization in the corpora cavernosa of the clitoris is essentially similar to that of the penis except for the absence of the subalguineal layer interposed between the tunica albuginea and erectile tissue" (Toesca, Stolfi, et al., 1996).

What these investigators concluded is that the anatomy of the clitoris is homologous (similar in form) to that of the penis and that in physical arousal it does everything that the penis does on a smaller, but no less important, scale. It follows that both male and female sexual organs are similarly affected by cardiovascular condition.

A PILL PROBLEM

Unfortunately, the drugs commonly used to treat hypertension—as well as those that lower cholesterol and protect against heart attacks, strokes, and atherosclerosis—can also negatively affect sexual function. This is particularly a problem when these drugs must be used in high doses. Sexual side effects and other problems with these drugs have led to the development of newer antihypertensive medications that are less likely to induce sexual side effects, and we encourage patients experiencing problems to discuss their issues with their physicians.

For many patients, simple dietary changes could help them lower their blood pressure and potentially lower their drug dosage.

Medications That Can Affect Sexual Function

What Is Sexual Dysfunction?

Sexual dysfunction refers to a problem during any phase of the sexual response cycle that prevents the individual or couple from experiencing satisfaction from the sexual activity. The sexual response cycle has four phases: excitement, plateau, orgasm, and resolution. Sexual dysfunction can be caused by physical and emotional factors, or a combination of both. The side effects of some medications can also lead to sexual dysfunction.

What Are the Types of Sexual Dysfunction?

Sexual dysfunction is generally classified into four categories:

- Desire disorders. The lack of sexual desire or interest in sex.
- Arousal disorders. The inability to become physically aroused during sexual activity, including problems achieving and maintaining an erection (erectile dysfunction).
- Orgasm disorders. The delay or absence of orgasm (climax).
- Pain disorders. Pain during intercourse (This mostly affects women.).

What Medications Can Cause Sexual Dysfunction?

Some prescription medications and even over-the-counter drugs can have an impact on sexual functioning. Some medicines can affect libido (desire) and others can affect the ability to become aroused or achieve orgasm. The risk of sexual side effects is increased when an individual is taking multiple medications.

Sexual side effects have been reported with the following medications:

Some over-the-counter antihistamines and decongestants can cause erectile dysfunction or problems with ejaculation.

ANTIDEPRESSANTS

- Tricyclic antidepressants, including amitriptyline (Elavil), doxepin (Sinequan), imipramine (Tofranil), and nortriptyline (Aventyl, Pamelor).

- Monoamine oxidase inhibitors (MAOIs), including phenelzine (Nardil) and tranylcypromine (Parnate).

- Anti-psychotic medications, including thiordiazine (Mellaril), thiothixene (Navane), and haloperidol (Haldol).

- Anti-mania medications such as lithium carbonate (Eskalith, Lithobid).

- Selective serotonin reuptake inhibitors (SSRIs) such as fluoxetine (Prozac), sertraline (Zoloft), and paroxetine (Paxil).

ANTI-HYPERTENSIVE MEDICATIONS (USED TO TREAT HIGH BLOOD PRESSURE)

- Diuretics, including spironolactone (Aldactone) and the thiazides (Diuril, Naturetin, and others).

- Centrally acting agents, including methyldopa (Aldomet) and reserpine (Serpasil, Raudixin).

- α-Adrenergic (alpha) blockers, including prazosin (Minipress) and terazosin (Hytrin).

- β-Adrenergic (beta) blockers, including propranolol (Inderal) and metoprotol (Lopressor).

HORMONES

- Lupron.

- Zoladex.

Reproduced with permission from the Cleveland Clinic Foundation.

DEPRESSION AND DYSFUNCTION

When fluoxetine (Prozac) became available in the United States, it quickly became the most widely prescribed antidepressant ever to hit the marketplace. It seemed to have no significant adverse side effects, and its toxicity was low. The manufacturer reported a 1.9 percent incidence of sexual dysfunction complaints in controlled clinical trials. By 1990, however, reports of a higher incidence of sexual dysfunction began to emerge (Wagner, no date given).

A McGraw-Hill Companies website, Hospital Practice, now tells us that "Sexual dysfunction is a common side effect seen in patients taking selective serotonin reuptake inhibitors" (SSRIs). Prozac is the most commonly prescribed of these drugs, and sexual dysfunction contributed to a Prozac backlash (Moore and Rothschild, 1999). One undesirable effect of these drugs is anorgasmia, the failure to reach orgasm. Anorgasmia is often treated with—you guessed it—more drugs.

As we have seen, because sexual vitality depends on healthy blood vessels, many of the risk factors for sexual dysfunction in men and women are exactly the same as the risk factors for cardiovascular disease, heart disease, stroke, and diabetes: sedentary lifestyle, obesity, smoking tobacco, excessive alcohol consumption, and diets deficient in fresh fruits and vegetables and high in saturated fats (Derby, Mohr, et al., 2000). As our culture has evolved, our physical activity levels and diet have devolved, leaving us overweight, tired, and definitely not as sexy.

WHAT'S AGE GOT TO DO WITH IT?

> *It does not matter how slow you go, as long as you do not stop.*
>
> —CONFUCIUS

Many of us assume that the eroding desire for lovemaking that progresses with age is simply a natural, inevitable process. Although some research supports that sexual daydreaming and sexual drive decrease with aging, nearly 95 percent of the older people in one sample reported that they liked sex, and 75 percent reported that orgasm was important to their sexual fulfillment (Starr and Weiner, 1982). Although there are physical changes that occur with aging, sexual activity is influenced by psychological well-being, depth of intimacy, and cultural expectations.

An active sexual expression of physical pleasure (whether or not intercourse is included) does not necessarily decrease as we age. Research suggests that the best predictor of future sexual satisfaction is past performance. This means that the sooner you get into a regular pattern of pleasurable sex, the more likely it is to continue throughout your life. A couple in their eighties succinctly described their attitude toward sex: "We feel it is much better to wear out than to rust out" (Brecker, 1984).

For many older adults, the greatest challenge (other than finding a suitable partner) is feeling that it is normal to enjoy sex well into their seventies and beyond! Many hide their sexual activities from friends and relatives, fearing disapproval. Masters and Johnson summed up the problem in 1981: "For some inexplicable reason, society has been uncomfortable with any overt expression of an active interest in sexual function by an older man or woman or unable to accept without reservation any aging person's demands for freedom to express his or her basic sexuality."

As intimacy increases, the capacity for passion increases. Couples in long-term relationships who have continued to work at developing their closeness and intimacy have the greatest potential for enjoying extraordinary sex.

What these studies show us is that sex is related to both health and happiness for people of all ages. An encouraging study from the AARP reported that for the majority of midlife and older adults (67 percent of men and 57 percent of women), a satisfying sexual relationship remains extremely important to quality of life. Even better, like fine wine, the percent who view their partners as romantic and/or physically attractive may actually increase with age.

For example, among men ages forty-five through seventy-four, 59 percent feel strongly that their partner is "physically attractive"; this increases to 63 percent when they are seventy-five or over. Fifty-two percent of women ages forty-five through fifty-nine feel this way about their partner, and the number increases to 57 percent for women seventy-five and older.

Many more older women find their partners romantic: 53 percent for women seventy-five or older versus only 29 percent ages forty-five through fifty-nine. (The AARP/*Modern Maturity* sexuality study was a mail survey of 1,384 adults ages forty-five and older, completed during March 1999, by NFO Research, Inc.)

Examining the sales growth of Viagra further refutes the notion that sexual activity inevitably declines with age: Viagra is prescribed annually in the United States to about twenty-three million men and enjoys sales of more than $1.5 billion. Since Viagra supports sexual *performance* and has no effect on sexual *desire,* the Viagra phenomenon gives strong evidence that the majority of men with sexual dysfunction strongly desire sex— enough to pay a considerable sum to enhance its performance.

We are now learning that this is also true for women: Lack of sexual vitality, previously called frigidity, is also often present in the face of strong desire.

The notion that low sexual vitality and inadequate, unsatisfying sexual performance stems from low desire is just not true for most people. For many of us, poor nutrition is the culprit, and a nutritional makeover is the solution.

Cardiovascular fitness, far more than age, is the crucial factor in sexual functioning. Medical science has now established that sexual vitality does not have to "naturally" deteriorate with time. In fact, the biological age of those who stay sexually active (and properly nourished) is many years younger than their chronological age.

Partners can retain their orgasmic enjoyment well into their advanced years. In women, many of the issues that can impact sexual pleasure respond positively to estrogen replacement therapy. Use of water-soluble lubricants (such as Astroglide) can help relieve vaginal dryness that can make intercourse uncomfortable.

Older men may experience a longer refractory period between erections, because, following orgasm, their erection subsides more quickly, and it takes longer to ejaculate again. Yet younger and older men report no difference in their level of sexual satisfaction or enjoyment (Schiavi, et al., 1990).

"Once I asked Grandma when you stop liking it, and she was eighty:

She said, 'Child, you'll have to ask someone older than me' " (Tavris and Sadd, 1977).

WOMEN'S ISSUES: FEMALE DYSFUNCTION EXPLAINED

In Kinsey's time (in the 1950s), about twice as many men as women said they didn't have sex often enough. Now as many women as men are likely to make that complaint. The good news for women, according to gynecologist Dr. Claire Bailey of the University of Bristol, is that there is little or no risk of a woman's overdosing on sex. In fact, she said, ". . . regular sessions can not only firm a woman's tummy and buttocks but also improve her posture."

As with men who can suffer prostate enlargement as a consequence of not having sex, women who abstain from sex also run some risks. Particularly in postmenopausal women, vaginal atrophy can occur. This condition can lead to dyspareunia, or pain associated with intercourse, creating a vicious cycle of avoiding sex. In addition, women who fail to climax may find sex less appealing, and the less sex they have, the more difficult it can become to ever experience orgasm.

For women without a sexual partner, some doctors advocate use of a vibrator to maintain vaginal function. Vibrators can also make it easier for many women to have an orgasm, and can improve enjoyment of sex with or without a partner.

The "Report of the International Consensus Development Conference on Female Sexual Dysfunction: Definitions and Classifications" explained:

> Female sexual dysfunction is a multicausal and multidimensional problem combining biological, psychological and interpersonal determinants. It is age-related, progressive and highly prevalent, affecting 20% to 50% of women. Based on epidemiological data from the National Health and Social Life Survey, a third of women lack sexual interest and nearly a fourth do not experience orgasm. (Laumann, Paik, et al., 1999). Approximately 20% of women report lubrication difficulties and 20% find sex not pleasurable. Female sexual dysfunction has a major impact on quality of life and interpersonal relationships. For

many women it has been physically disconcerting, emotionally distressing and socially disruptive.

In contrast to the widespread interest in research and treatment of male sexual dysfunction, less attention has been paid to sexual problems of women. Few studies have investigated the psychological and physiological underpinnings of female sexual dysfunction and fewer treatments are available for women than for men. A major barrier to the development of clinical research and practice has been the absence of a well-defined, broadly accepted diagnostic framework and classification for female sexual dysfunction. [Basson, Berman, et al., 2000]

HOW DO WE DEFINE FSD?

Sexual dysfunction is defined as disturbances in sexual desire and in the psycho-physiological changes that characterize the sexual response cycle and cause marked distress and interpersonal difficulty.

The female sexual response cycle consists of three phases: desire, arousal, and orgasm. Various organs of the external and internal genitalia, including vagina, clitoris, labia minora, vestibular bulbs, pelvic floor muscles, and uterus, contribute to female sexual function. During sexual arousal, genital blood flow and sensation are increased. The vaginal canal is moistened (lubrication). During orgasm, there is rhythmical contraction of the uterus and pelvic floor muscles.

Sexual arousal largely depends on the sympathetic nervous system, and various hormones may influence female sexual function. Estrogens have a significant role in maintaining vaginal mucosal epithelium as well as sensory thresholds and genital blood flow. Androgens primarily affect sexual desire, arousal, orgasm, and the overall sense of well-being.

As noted on page 13, the model for female sexual function has morphed from a linear, causal model to a circular one. In a similar way, we must also reexamine our definitions of FSD. We have come a long way from the days when women with sexual dysfunction were labeled "frigid," a term describing a subconscious distaste for engaging in sex with men.

An archived article from Harvard Medical School's *Harvard Health*

Publication has raised some very cogent points suggesting the possibility that we may be trying to rearrange the spots on the leopard with regard to definitions of FSD. The article pointed out that female sexual function is qualitative, not quantitative, compared with that in men. This raises the question: What qualifies as dysfunctional?

The American Foundation for Urologic Disease has been trying on a yearly basis to mirror the work of a National Institutes of Health panel that developed diagnostic and treatment guidelines for erectile dysfunction. Building on definitions of sexual dysfunction from the World Health Organization's International Classification of Diseases (ICD-10), focusing on physical factors and the American Psychiatric Association's Diagnostic and Statistical Manual of Mental Disorders (DSM-IV-R), focusing on psychological factors, the Foundation's first report (in the March 2000 issue of the *Journal of Urology*) proposed a working definition of sexual dysfunction in women that includes both physiological and psychological symptoms (see the Female Sexual Function Index sidebar). Experiencing any one of them warrants an FSD diagnosis, but must also be a source of "distress" for the woman in order to qualify as a sign of FSD.

Female Sexual Function Index [*†‡]

1. Over the past 4 weeks how often did you experience discomfort during sexual intercourse?
    _____Did not attempt sexual intercourse
    _____Almost always or always
    _____Most times (much more than half the time)
    _____Sometimes (about half the time)
    _____A few times (much less than half the time)
    _____Almost never or never

2. Over the past 4 weeks how often did you experience dryness during sexual intercourse?
    _____Did not attempt sexual intercourse
    _____Almost always or always

_____Most times (much more than half the time)

_____Sometimes (about half the time)

_____A few times (much less than half the time)

_____Almost never or never

3. Over the past 4 weeks how often did you attempt sexual intercourse?

   _____0

   _____1–2

   _____3–4

   _____5–6

   _____7–10

   _____11+

4. Over the past 4 weeks how often have you felt *sexual desire*?

   _____Almost never/never

   _____A few times (much less than half the time)

   _____Sometimes (about half the time)

   _____Most times (much more than half the time)

   _____Almost always/always

5. Over the past 4 weeks how would you rate your level of *sexual desire*?

   _____Very low/none at all

   _____Low

   _____Moderate

   _____High

   _____Very high

6. Over the past 4 weeks how satisfied have you been with your overall *sex life*?

   _____Very dissatisfied

   _____Moderately dissatisfied

   _____About equally satisfied and dissatisfied

   _____Moderately satisfied

   _____Very satisfied

7. Over the past 4 weeks how satisfied have you been with your *sexual relationship* with your partner?

_____Very dissatisfied

_____Moderately dissatisfied

_____About equally satisfied and dissatisfied

_____Moderately satisfied

_____Very satisfied

8. Over the past 4 weeks, when you had sexual stimulation *or* intercourse, how often did you have the feeling of orgasm?

_____Almost never/never

_____A few times (much less than half the time)

_____Sometimes (about half the time)

_____Most times (much more than half the time)

_____Almost always/always

9. Over the past 4 weeks, when you had sexual stimulation *or* intercourse, how would you rate your degree of *clitoral sensation*?

_____Very low/none at all

_____Low

_____Moderate

_____High

_____Very high

---

*Sexual function includes intercourse, caressing, foreplay, and masturbation.
†Sexual intercourse is defined as vaginal penetration by your partner. (You were entered by your partner.)
‡Sexual stimulation includes situations like foreplay with a partner, looking at erotic pictures, etc.

From Kaplan, Reis, et al., 1999. Reprinted with permission from Elsevier.

While it is now clear that FSD is also a medical problem, the "pharmacy" for women, unlike that for men, is compounded by hormonal changes that take place as they age.

The major complaints of women with FSD are loss of interest in sex, vaginal dryness (failure to lubricate and engorge the vagina and the clitoris with even "adequate" stimulation), and pain during intercourse. These components are presumed to be independent of one another. For instance, someone with decreased sexual desire may still be capable of arousal and orgasm.

There is a strong link between advancing age and decreased clitoral cavernosal smooth-muscle fibers: Aging women undergo changes in clitoral cavernosal erectile tissue that may play an as-yet-undetermined role in age-associated female sexual dysfunction (Connell, Guess, et al., 2005).

It is more problematic to track age-related circulating levels of sex hormones in women than in men because there are more than thirty different forms of estrogen, their blood concentration varies over the menstrual cycle, and the blood levels drop precipitously and rapidly at menopause. Conventional "reference range" information used by physicians to evaluate circulating hormone concentrations tells us that postmenopausal levels are about the same as prepuberty levels: less than 40 pg/ml. At its greatest concentration on the twelfth day of the menstrual cycle, the reference range for estradiol is 156 to 437 pg/ml.

A Question of Desire

> *Some desire is necessary to keep life in motion.*
>
> —SAMUEL JOHNSON

Loss of sexual desire, also known as hypoactive sexual desire (HSDD), is now fast becoming one of the more common complaints that women of all ages report to their ob-gyn physicians. An estimated one-third of women between the ages of eighteen and fifty-nine complain of lost interest in sex, according to Drs. J. Warner and B. Nazario. Unlike men's principal complaint of erectile dysfunction, women's loss of sexual desire is not likely to be cured with a pill.

The medical and psychological communities do not reject altogether the idea that there are many individuals who suffer from sexual dysfunction because of a lack of desire (libido). Increasingly, though, cardiovascular function and hormone levels are thought to account for this decline in interest.

Sexual desire decreases with age in women because, unlike men, the body undergoes a biological change in sex-driving hormones including androgens: While estrogens maintain the response to sexual stimulation, lubrication, and engorgement, testosterone drives desire (Berman, Berman, et al., 1999). Testosterone affects sexual drive in both men and women. Testosterone levels peak in women's midtwenties and then steadily decline until menopause, when they drop dramatically. But Drs. Warner and Nazario caution that hormones are unlikely to play the only role in HSD and that there are a number of common causes:

• **Interpersonal relationship issues.** These include partner performance problems, lack of emotional satisfaction with the relationship, birth of a child, and becoming a caregiver for a loved one.

• **Sociocultural influences.** Job stress, peer pressure, and media images of sexuality can negatively influence sexual desire.

• **Age.** Blood levels of androgens fall continuously as women age.

• **Medical problems.** Mental illnesses, such as depression, or medical conditions, like endometriosis, fibroids, and thyroid disorders, impact a woman's sexual drive both mentally and physically.

• **Medications.** Certain antidepressants (including the new generation of SSRIs), blood-pressure-lowering drugs, and oral contraceptives can lower sexual drive in many ways, such as decreasing available testosterone levels or affecting blood flow (tables 2.1 and 2.2).

TABLE 2.1

Medications Associated with Female Sexual Dysfunction

Antihistamines	Antiandrogens	Alcohol
Sympathomimetic amines	Cimetidine	Antiestrogens
Anticonvulsants	Spironolactone	Tamoxifen
Metronidazole	Alkylating agents	Raloxifen
Metoclopramide	Cyclophosphamide	Gonadotropin-
Antihypertensives	Anticholinergics	releasing
Diuretics	Oral contraceptives	hormone
Adrenergic antagonists	Drugs with abuse	analgesics
(terazosin, doxazosin)	potential	(leuprolide,
β-Blockers	Antidepressants	goserelin)
Calcium channel	Hypnotics	
blockers	Sedatives	

From Lightner, D. J. Female Sexual Dysfunction. *Mayo Clinic Proceedings.* 2002; 77:698–702. Reprinted with permission.

TABLE 2.2

Medications that May Cause Female Sexual Dysfunction

Anti-hypertensives	Anti-depressants	Anxiolytics	Illicit and Abused Drugs	Miscellaneous
benazepril (Lotensin)	amoxapine (Asendin)	alprazolam (Xanax)	alcohol	acetazolamide (Diamox)
clonidine (Catapres)	bupropion (Wellbutrin, Wellbutrin SR, Zyban)	barbiturates	amphetamines	amiodarone (Cordarone, Pacerone)
lisinopril (Prinivil, Zestril)	buspirone (BuSpar)	clomipramine (Anafranil)	amyl nitrate	bromocriptine (Parlodel)
methyldopa (Aldomet)	fluoxetine (Prozac, Sarafem)	clonazepam (Klonopin)	barbiturates	cimetidine (Tagamet)
metoprolol (Lopressor, Toprol XL)	imipramine (Tofranil)	diazepam (Valium, Diastat)	cocaine	danazol (Danocrine)
propranolol (Inderal, Inderal LA)	paroxetine (Paxil)	lithium (Eskalith, Eskalith CR, Lithobid, Lithonate)	diazepam (Valium, Diastat)	digoxin (Lanoxin, Digitek, Lanoxicaps)
reserpine (Serpasil)	phenelzine (Nardil)	lorazepam (Ativan)	marijuana	diphenhydramine (Benadryl)
spironolactone (Aldactone)	sertraline (Zoloft)	perphenazine (Trilafon)	MDMA (ecstasy, methylmethylenedioxyamphetamine)	ethinyl estradiol (Estinyl, FemHRT, various oral contraceptives)
timolol (Blocadren)	trazodone (Desyrel) venlafaxine (Effexor)	prochlorperazine (Compazine)	morphine tobacco	gemfibrozil (Lopid) medroxyprogesterone (Amen, Cycrin, Depo-Provera, Provera) metronidazole (Flagyl) niacin (Niacor, Niaspan) phenytoin (Dilantin) ranitidine (Zantac)

Reproduced with permission from the Cleveland Clinic Foundation.

Diagnosing HSDD

Obtaining a valid diagnosis of FSD can be a daunting process. Often a detailed history is followed by a physical examination and extensive laboratory studies. Physiological monitoring of reaction to arousal potentially allows diagnosis of organic diseases where there is measurable deficiency. Duplex Doppler sonography and photoplethysmography (the measurement of vaginal and minor labial blood vessel oxygen concentration) may help to evaluate genital blood flow. Moreover, measurements of vaginal pH and compliance should be performed.

Neurophysiological examination—such as measurement of the bulbocavernosus reflex and pudendal evoked potentials; of genital sympathetic skin response (SSR); and of warm, cold, and vibratory perception thresholds, as well as testing of the pressure and touch sensitivity of the external genitalia—should be performed to evaluate neurogenic etiologies. All this, of course, requires the attention of a specialist ob-gyn physician.

A number of treatments suggested by Drs. Warner and Nazario include sex therapy and relationship counseling, readjusting medications, addressing existing medical conditions that may contribute to HSDD, and considering varying ways of supplementing estrogens (such as in vaginal creams) and testosterone (as in patches).

Nonpharmacological Therapy for HSDD: Kegel Exercises

Biofeedback-type exercises were initially developed by a surgeon, Dr. Arnold Kegel, for the strengthening of anal or urinary sphincter muscles damaged in surgery, as part of treatment for incontinence: the perineometer consisted of a cone-shaped, flexible rubber chamber attached to a length of slender rubber tubing that led to a pressure gauge—the "feedback" device. The rubber chamber was inserted into the anus or vagina; by trial and error, contractions of the sphincter or outer vaginal muscles were noted as pressure changes on the gauge, reflecting the strength of the contractions.

The device and method have been adapted to train the vaginal pubococcygeus muscle, since it has been determined that exercising this muscle improves chances of attaining orgasm in anorgasmic women. Typical resting pressure, about 5 mm/Hg, can be raised to about 15 mm/Hg by contractions of the muscles (Levitt, Konovsky, et al., 1979).

Sexual Pharmacology for Women with HSDD

We have seen that hormones, primarily testosterone, that drive desire do not decline significantly with age in men. But hormones do decline significantly with age in women, and this decrease can depress desire. This fact may help explain why trials of Viagra in women have been inconclusive: The problem for women is not inhibiting PDE5, but stimulating the ACh-NO-cGMP sequence in the first place.

For some women, loss of desire may improve with hormone therapy, and they should not hesitate to discuss their lack of desire with their physicians. A new testosterone patch not yet approved by the Food and Drug Administration (FDA) appears promising for the treatment of HSDD. Procter & Gamble Pharmaceuticals, which manufactures the testosterone patch, plans to market it as Intrinsa if it is approved by the FDA.

In a recent clinical study presented at the Endocrine Society's Eighty-sixth Annual Meeting in New Orleans, researchers reported the effects of the patch in a twenty-four-week, randomized, double-blind, multicenter study. The study consisted of 447 surgically menopausal women receiving oral estrogen, who reported low sexual desire that caused distress. Patients received a placebo patch or a transdermal testosterone patch designed to deliver 150, 300, or 450 micrograms (μg) of testosterone per day. All patches were changed twice weekly.

The primary efficacy target of the study was the frequency of satisfying sexual activity as recorded in a Sexual Activity Log (SAL), and the sexual desire domain of the Profile of Female Sexual Function (PFSF), a multinational, validated instrument that measures seven domains of sexual function: desire, arousal, orgasm, pleasure, responsiveness, concerns, and self-image.

The group treated with the 300-μg/day testosterone patch experienced a 30 percent increase in the frequency of total satisfying sexual activity versus the placebo group, and an 81 percent increase versus baseline at twenty-four weeks. The 150-μg/day group was similar to placebo; no advantage of the 450-μg/day group over the 300-μg/day group was seen.

The 300-μg/day group also experienced a 66 percent increase in sexual desire versus baseline and a significant increase versus placebo. Dose-related increases in mean concentrations of free, total, and bioavailable testosterone were observed, and androgen concentrations significantly correlated with multiple PFSF and SAL domains.

Overall, adverse events (AE) reports were similar in the placebo and testosterone groups. The most common AEs reported were application site reactions, infection, acne, and headache.

A large-scale replication of this study with naturally menopausal women yielded just about the same results (Kroll, 2004). Since then, however, additional adverse "masculinizing" reactions have been noted, including facial hair growth.

Medical management of female sexual dysfunction so far is primarily based on hormone replacement therapy: Application of local estrogen can decrease pain and burning during intercourse. The efficacy of various other medications—sildenafil, arginine, yohimbine, phentolamine, apomorphine, and prostaglandin E1—in the treatment of female sexual dysfunction is still under investigation (Hilz and Marthol, 2004).

MEN'S ISSUES: MALE DYSFUNCTION EXPLAINED

In common terms, when things don't work for men, what's broken? The complaints take a number of different forms. In some cases, men may lose interest in sex, but that is not typically the case. Men more commonly complain of declining erectile strength and loss of sexual vigor. This usually means that erections may be reported to occur less reliably, to be less firm, perhaps to be less sustainable, and in some cases unattainable.

Differentiating between psychogenic (psychological/emotional) sources of erectile dysfunction (ED) and physiological, or medical, causes has often been problematic. To that end, Dutch researchers developed the aptly named Leiden Impotence Screening Test (LIST), alternatively known as the Leiden Impotence Questionnaire (LIQ). Though Leiden in the title refers to the Dutch city where the test was developed, ironically the word *leiden* in German means "to suffer." (If you would like to take the test, see table 2.3.)

TABLE 2.3

Leiden Impotence Questionnaire (LIQ): Items Differentiating Between Subjects with Organic and Those with Psychogenic ED

Items (shown according to groupings of questions in the LIQ)	Organic ED N=109 (%)	Psychogenic ED N=67 (%)	p*
General questions			
1. Financial problems	42 (38)	37 (56)	< 0.05
Current sexual functioning			
2. Sudden onset of ED	31 (28)	28 (42)	N.S.
3. Presence morning erections	76 (70)	59 (88)	< 0.01
4. Rigidity morning erections ≥ 50% of previous normal erections	40 (37)	44 (66)	< 0.01
5. Rigidity masturbatory erections ≥ 50% of previous normal erections	32 (29)	36 (54)	< 0.001
6. Rigidity coital erections ≥ 50% of previous normal erections	41 (38)	40 (60)	< 0.01
7. Adequate erections with different partner	3 (3)	7 (10)	< 0.05
8. Perceived contractions during orgasm	41 (38)	13 (19)	< 0.01
9. Premature ejaculation	35 (32)	38 (57)	< 0.01
Sexual functioning before onset of ED			
10. Frequency coitus > 1/month	88 (81)	45 (67)	< 0.01
11. Duration coitus > 10 minutes	22 (20)	25 (37)	< 0.05
12. Perceived contractions during orgasm	61 (56)	23 (34)	< 0.01
Consequences of ED			
13. Reduced size of penis	69 (63)	30 (45)	< 0.05
14. Decline in sexual interest	40 (37)	37 (55)	< 0.05
15. Partner regards patient as not being a real man	38 (35)	33 (49)	< 0.05
16. Tension in relationship	34 (31)	30 (45)	< 0.05
17. Thoughts about separation	23 (21)	9 (13)	N.S.

Items (shown according to groupings of questions in the LIQ)	Organic ED N=109 (%)	Psychogenic ED N=67 (%)	p*
Patient's opinion about the cause of ED			
18. Psychogenic aetiology	30 (28)	35 (52)	< 0.01
19. Associated with psychological problems	38 (35)	45 (67)	< 0.001

*Chi-square tests.

Reprinted from Speckens, Hengveld, et al., 1993, with permission from Elsevier.

Some key differentiators that are an important part of diagnosing and treating erectile dysfunction, or ED, include:

• **Misattribution of low desire.** Men may quite understandably misinterpret ED as a reduced level of sexual desire (low libido). Indeed, ED can ultimately lead to loss of desire, because men may avoid sexual contact in order to avoid facing the possibility of ED.

• **Premature ejaculation.** Orgasmic dysfunction such as premature ejaculation (PE) is fairly common, but it has to be differentiated from ED. The term *PE* was changed to *rapid ejaculation (RE)* at the Second International Consultation on Erectile and Sexual Dysfunctions, held in Paris in June 2003. It should be noted that men with RE often refer to their condition as ED because there is a rapid loss of erection following RE.

• **Absent or delayed ejaculation.** Absent or delayed ejaculation requires a careful description. Is the problem only present with the partner or also when one is masturbating? Does it occur intravaginally or also outside the vagina?

• **Psychosocial history.** Psychosocial factors have been shown to interfere with satisfying sexual performance. These may include issues about self-esteem and social and occupational adjustment and performance, financial security, and family life. Stress either at home or on the job, or relating to social position satisfaction, along with education and lifestyle factors can all play a role in male sexual performance.

The Penile Nocturnal Tumescence Sign

The most important factor discriminating between psychogenic ED and organic ED in the Leiden studies was presence and rigidity of morning erections (items 3 and 4 on table 2.3).

Evidence of erection at night—typically toward morning—known as penile nocturnal tumescence, strongly suggests that the plumbing is basically sound and that the condition may well be readily treatable. This sign is not, however, a substitute for a medical diagnosis.

What About Testosterone?

Most men probably think that loss of sexual vitality is due to age-related declining testosterone levels. After all, other factors being equal, sex in both men and women is driven in large part by testosterone. But downward-spiraling testosterone levels as men age is largely a myth.

In figure 2.1, blood levels of testosterone in men are observed to rise over the first half of the average life span, to peak at about age forty. Then levels decline steadily, but very slowly, to well into the late seventies.

Note that testosterone levels at age seventy are about the same as they are at age twenty. Numerous medical reports corroborate these findings: Blood serum testosterone levels don't decline significantly until a man is well into his late seventies (Nawata, Kato, and Ibayashi, 1977). However, figure 2.1 shows only blood testosterone (T) levels—and that's not the whole male hormone story.

At about the time in a man's life when the testosterone levels are beginning to decline, the body converts some of it to a super-testosterone form, 5-alpha-dihydrotestosterone (5DHT). This fact is rarely mentioned in connection with age-related testosterone levels in men and, of course, it is not reflected in the figure.

It is 5DHT that causes pattern baldness beginning in a man's mid to late forties and early fifties. It also promotes the nettlesome prostate swelling that in many men leads to benign prostate hypertrophy (BPH), which can interfere with sexual vitality and can lead to prostate cancer in some men.

The same prescription medication used to inhibit the enzyme 5-alpha-reductase that converts testosterone to 5DHT, finasteride (Propecia), is used to treat pattern baldness and BPH. A popular herbal alternative to prescription medication, *Serenoa repens* (saw palmetto), as well as the mineral zinc have been medically proven to inhibit 5-alpha-reductase (Buck, 2004; Dvorkin and Song, 2002). But as with any other treatment, an appropriate medical expert should be consulted.

The production of testosterone declines very gradually from about 84 ng/ml in the twenty-to-forty age range, to about 79 ng/ml in the forty-to-sixty range, and finally to about 67 ng/ml among those sixty to eighty. This represents a decrease of only 20 percent from start to finish (Lewis, Ghanadian, et al., 1976). As you will see, the decline in hormone production in women undergoing menopause is considerably steeper.

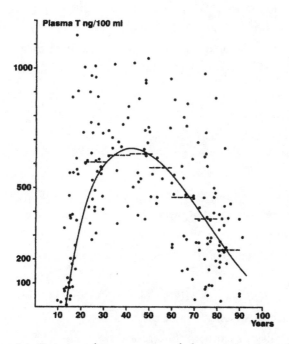

Figure 2.1: Variation of concentration of plasma testosterone (free and bound) with age in normal men. From Wagner, and Green, 1981. With permisson from Springer Verlag GmbH.

Diagnosing ED

There are, of course, instances when men experience ED as a direct result of medical problems. In some cases, it may have a basis in our nervous system—so-called neurogenic impotence (Hilz and Marthol, 2003). More commonly, it is a problem with our blood vessels—so-called vasculogenic impotence—specifically with the endothelium, as noted earlier (Chaitlin, 2004; Kaiser, Billups, et al., 2004). Table 2.4 classifies the medical causes of male sexual dysfunction.

Sexual Pharmacology for Men

The preferred medical treatment for ED today is the prescription of one or another of the phosphodiesterase type 5 (PDE5) inhibitors such as Viagra, Levitra, and Cialis. However, these tend to lower blood pressure—a side effect that could be hazardous for those also taking blood-pressure-lowering medications, including nitrates. As with any treatment, proper medical supervision is necessary. Some of the medical mishaps with these drugs have occurred as a result of using medication prescribed for a friend or family member without appropriate screening by a physician.

APHRODISIA

The reportedly successful use of yohimbine to treat low sexual desire in men was extended to the treatment of hypoactive sexual desire in women at the University of Mississippi Medical Center in Jackson. Nine women with hypoactive sex drives and a lower concentration of the blood factor MHPG (3-methoxy-4-hydroxyphenylglycol) were prescribed 5.4 mg/day orally of yohimbine hydrochloride, and then compared with seven controls.

Despite measurable plasma MHPG increase in the nine women with hypoactive sex drives, no measurable subjective change in sexual desire was noted as a result of treatment (Piletz, Segraves, et al., 1998).

SEXUAL HEALING AND THE THREE FOOD FACTORS

Sex is one of the nine reasons for incarnation. The other eight are unimportant.

—GEORGE BURNS

An inadequate diet can affect a person's sexual functioning in two ways. First, if the foods in the diet do not provide the nutrients to produce sufficient NO, the mechanism of erection, or engorgement in women, will be impaired. Second, if a high-fat diet has promoted atherosclerosis, the endothelium lining the sex organs may be damaged so that it cannot respond to ACh with the proper sequence of enzymes needed in the NO-cGMP sequence that causes erection.

Our plan, based on the three Food Factors—Greens and Beans (nitrogen-rich foods), Staminators (arginine sources), and the Brights (antioxidants)—addresses this dilemma in several ways. First, it provides nitrogen-rich and arginine-rich food sources of NO. Ingestion of nitrogen-rich foods can prevent the immediate adverse impact of a high-fat meal and increase the production of nitric oxide (Plotnick, Corretti, et al., 2003).

Second, the high-ORAC (see page 109), super-antioxidant-rich foods protect the endothelium from free radical damage. In some people, a diet high in antioxidants can even reverse the accumulation of the damaging atherosclerotic plaque formation so that the endothelium can function again to respond to ACh. One medical journal reported, "In general, a 'prudent diet,' characterized by higher intake of fruits, vegetables, legumes, fish, poultry, and whole grains, is associated with a beneficial effect on the endothelium" (Lopez-Garcia and Hu, 2003).

Finally, age-related progressive impairment of the endothelium, even in individuals older than seventy, can be improved by arginine (Bode-Boger, Muke, et al., 2003).

As recent medical science confirms, cardiovascular health has an immediate effect on sexual functioning. A high level of total cholesterol and a low level of HDL cholesterol are important risk factors in erectile dysfunction (Wei, Macera, et al., 1994). In fact, cardiovascular risk factors predict erectile dysfunction (Sullivan, Miller, et al., 2001).

TABLE 2.4

Causes of Sexual Dysfunction in the Male Classified by Clinical Manifestation

Clinical manifestation	Most common causes
Disorders of desire	
Hypoactive sexual desire (HSD)	Psychogenic (e.g., depression, marital discord leading to desire deficiency, performance anxiety leading to excitement inhibition)
	CNS disease (partial epilepsy, Parkinson's, poststroke, adrenoleukodystrophy)
	Androgen deficiency (primary or secondary), androgen resistance
	Drugs (antihypertensives, psychotropics, alcohol, narcotics, dopamine blockers, antiandrogens)
Compulsive sexual behaviors	Psychogenic (obsessive-compulsive sexuality, excessive sex-seeking in association with affective disorders, addictive sexuality, sex impulsivity)
Erectile dysfunction	Psychogenic
	Drugs (antihypertensives, anticholinergics, psychotropics, cigarette smoking, substance abuse)
	Systemic diseases (cardiac, hepatic, renal, pulmonary, cancer, metabolic, post–organ transplant, pelvic irradiation)
	Androgen deficiency (primary or secondary), androgen resistance, other endocrinopathics
	Vascular insufficiency (atherosclerosis, pelvic steal, penile Raynaud's, venous leakage)
	Neurological disorder (Parkinson's, Alzheimer's, Shy-Drager, encephalopathy, spinal cord or nerve injury)
	Penile disease (Peyronie's, priapism, phimosis, smooth muscle dysfunction, trauma)
Disorders of ejaculation	
Premature ejaculation (primary or secondary)	Psychogenic (neurotic personality, anxiety/depression, partner discord or other situational factors)

Clinical manifestation	Most common causes
Premature ejaculation (cont'd)	Organic (increased central dopaminergic activity, increased penile sensitivity)
Absent or retarded emission	Sympathetic denervation (diabetes, surgical injury, irradiation)
	Drugs (sympatholytics, CNS depressants)
	Androgen deficiency (primary or secondary), androgen resistance
Postejaculation pain	Psychogenic
Orgasmic dysfunction	Drugs (selective serotonin reuptake inhibitors, tricyclic antidepressants, monoamine oxidase inhibitors, substance abuse)
	CNS disease (multiple sclerosis, Parkinson's, Huntington's chorea, lumbar sympathectomy)
	Psychogenic (performance anxiety, conditioning factors, fear of impregnation, hypoactive sexual desire)
Failure of detumescence	
Structural penile disease	Penile structural abnormalities (Peyronie's, phimosis)
Priapism (primary or secondary)	Primary priapism: idiopathic
	Priapism secondary to disease: hematologic (sickle cell anemia, leukemia, multiple myeloma), infiltrative (Fabry's disease, amyloidosis), inflammatory (tularemia, mumps), and neurologic diseases, solid tumors, trauma
	Priapism secondary to drugs: phenothiazines, trazodone, cocaine, intrapenile vasoactive injections

From: Kandeel, F. R., Koussa, V. K. T., and R. S. Swerdloff (2001): Male sexual function and its disorders: Physiology, pathophysiology, clinical investigation, and treatment. *Endocrine Reviews*, 22, 342–388. Adapted from Swerdloff, R. S., and F. R. Kandeel (1992): *Textbook of Internal Medicine*. Philadelphia: Lippincott Williams & Wilkins Co. Reprinted with permission.

As noted earlier, hyperlipidemia (elevated serum cholesterol) is common in men with erectile dysfunction. The ratio of total cholesterol (TC) to HDL cholesterol (HDL-C)—TC/HDL-C—predicts erectile dysfunction: "Erectile dysfunction might therefore serve as a sentinel event for coronary heart disease" (Roumegerre, Wespes, et al., 2003). Improving cardiovascular heart risks, especially lipid-lowering strategies, in midlife may decrease the risk of erectile dysfunction (Fung, Bettencourt, et al., 2004).

TO MARKET AND THEN TO BED

Culturally, we tend to divide the body into two segments: above the waist and below the waist. Above the waist, the cardiovascular system (CVS) consists of the heart, which pumps blood under pressure through a closed, flexible system of conduits or blood vessels (vas) to all parts of the body and the brain. The blood vessels leaving the heart branch off, and the branches diminish in diameter more or less as they become more distant from the heart and serve its different organs.

The real story is that the body is connected above and below the waist by the same circulatory system. Therefore, the same diet that clogs the vessels of your heart can ultimately impair blood flow to your sexual organs. This is why we like to refer to our internal plumbing as the cardiosexual system.

Let us be perfectly clear: *Great Food, Great Sex* does not claim to make you want more sex, but it will help you to have better sex when you do want it. In terms of human behavior, a pleasant experience is more rewarding than an unpleasant one—the more often you have pleasurable sex, the more likely you will be to want to repeat the experience.

For those fortunate men and women among you who do not experience sexual dysfunction, *Great Food, Great Sex* can safeguard your sex life. Our three Food Factors provide high-octane fuel to maintain top-level sexual vitality and performance.

You can use *Great Food, Great Sex* to help you evaluate your own state of health. We urge you to try our program for six short weeks, and see what a difference a diet can make.

3

The Science Behind the Great Food, Great Sex Plan

The Miracle Molecule NO

The most important sex organ is the brain. Thinking about sex leads to arousal for most people. This makes sense considering what we understand to be the role of chemicals and neurotransmitters in the sexual cascade. The message gets from above the neck to below the belt by way of a series of chemical reactions that are conveyed through the bloodstream to different parts of the body by neurotransmitters. Simply put, blood vessels need to be kept open or the messages don't get through.

Some time ago, science tracked down acetylcholine (ACh), the first level of neurotransmitter associated with sexual desire that leaves the brain and travels through the bloodstream to the sex organs. More recently, we discovered a critically important chemical associated with sexual arousal—an unexpected go-between neurotransmitter. It is a simple two-atom gas molecule, nitric oxide (NO), made by the endothelium that lines the arterial blood vessels, as well as by the insides of the sexual organs.

Great Food, Great Sex optimizes sexual health by outlining a nutritional method for supplying the body with an adequate supply of nitric oxide—the essential fuel for peak sexual performance—and by ensuring the health of the endothelium tissues that respond to it.

The recent discovery of the crucial biological role of NO unlocked an important mystery of sexual function. NO is a gas that the body extracts from many common foods, and NO controls the key enzymes necessary to sexual function. When your body is sexually stimulated, the brain sends out the chemical messenger ACh to the blood vessels in the sex organs. ACh activates a series of enzymes that cause the endothelium to extract NO from the bloodstream. NO causes the blood vessels to open up—dilate—thus increasing blood flow.

Without an adequate supply of NO circulating in the bloodstream, sexual vitality declines and aging accelerates. Medical experts now recognize that the combination of low NO production and damaged endothelium cells can cause bedroom performance issues for both men and women.

IT'S YOUR PLATE, NOT YOUR MATE

The only readily available source of NO in the body is the food you consume. Many common foods are excellent sources of NO, but the typical American diet of highly processed, preserved, low-fiber foods, high in refined carbohydrates (sugar) and saturated fats, is not NO-friendly.

Americans consume about one-third of their daily caloric intake as junk food containing high levels of saturated fats and refined sugars. Our poor eating habits compromise our sexual health in two ways. First, the foods that could supply adequate NO are often noticeably missing from our high-fat, low-vegetable, low-fruit diets. Second, this nutritionally deficient diet impairs the ability of the vessels to respond to NO, by causing damage to the endothelium.

Blood vessels are alive: They breathe, they eat, they move, they constrict, and they expand. What's more, they have to do this in the right location at the right time. Blood vessels depend on NO to transport crucial chemical messages to various parts of the body.

One sure way to short-circuit these messages is to insult the vessels with oxidized LDL-cholesterol-forming atherosclerotic plaque. Plaque is a deposit of cholesterol combined with a variant—free radical—form of oxygen to which has been added immune system cell debris and calcium. Cholesterol will invariably oxidize this way in the presence of free radicals.

Free radicals are generated primarily by many of the foods we eat, our metabolism, and activity including vigorous exercise. When plaque forms inside the wall of an artery, it essentially narrows the channel through which blood can flow because the wall swells inward, encroaching into the lumen, the space through which blood flows. Atherosclerotic plaque is the very nemesis of bedroom fun.

Our high consumption of salty processed foods not only contributes to the high blood pressure of nearly thirty million people in this country, but also impairs sexual function. *Great Food, Great Sex* provides an alternative approach to obtaining adequate levels of NO—and improving its ability to work—through a combination of specific dietary nutrients:

- Nitrogen compounds, which we call Greens and Beans.

- Arginine, which we call Staminators.

- Super antioxidants, which we call the Brights.

These nutrients comprise the *three Food Factors for sexual fitness*. The three Food Factors of *Great Food, Great Sex* work in concert to enhance and restore sexual fitness by improving the health of your blood vessels, your cardiovascular system, and your heart. Just as distance runners adjust the composition of their diet to keep going for the long race, you can change your eating habits and reap the benefits in bed.

For those readers interested in a comprehensive understanding of the scientific mechanisms upon which the plan is based, a more detailed history follows.

SEX AND THE SCIENTISTS

Medicine has long known that ACh relaxes the smooth muscles that make up our arterial blood vessels. But a further discovery about ACh occurred in the laboratory of Dr. R. Furchgott at SUNY Downstate Medical College, Brooklyn, New York (Furchgott and Zawadzki, 1990). It provided a key to unlocking the mystery of sexual function, and ultimately to the foods that promote its vigorous performance.

The arterial vascular system of your body is made up of arteries, arterioles, and capillaries that transport oxygenated blood from the lungs to all parts of the body. The blood is pumped to the various locations under pressure by the heart. The blood vessels look much like pipes or tubes, distinguished principally by differences in diameter, going from larger arteries to virtually microscopic capillaries. Blood returns to the lungs, where excess carbon dioxide is eliminated and fresh oxygen is absorbed, and it courses also through the kidneys, where the waste products of metabolism are eliminated. The process is circular and continuous.

We also tend to think of our blood vessels as pipes like those that deliver water to the kitchen sink. But if you look at them under a microscope, they are in fact made up of a tubular structure consisting of adjacent endothelial cells, one cell thick. This tubular sheet of endothelial cells, the endothelium, is surrounded by overlapping rings of living smooth-muscle cells arranged in a way that forms and maintains the tubular shape of the blood vessel. These muscle rings can respond to chemical messages that cause them either to constrict, thus narrowing the vessel, or to relax, dilating it.

The chemical messengers are produced by the brain or by other body organs in response to activity needs, and they are commonly delivered to the blood vessel through the bloodstream. In some people, the arterial blood vessels throughout the body are chronically somewhat constricted by a continuous delivery of *constrict* messages. This impedes blood flow and causes the condition of elevated blood pressure we call hypertension.

Dr. Furchgott and colleagues were puzzling over the fact that the body's principal mechanism for lowering blood pressure, ACh, rarely works effectively for people with hypertension. A common model for studying the way that arterial blood vessels dilate or constrict is to examine a segment of the neck (carotid) artery of rabbits. Rabbit arteries respond to neurotransmitter substances in a fashion similar to our own response. In fact, deprived of their usual nitrate-rich diet (lots of greens and root vegetables), NO-donor foods, and instead fed our cholesterol-rich diet, rabbits quickly develop atherosclerosis.

Rabbit arteries should respond to ACh in the same way that our arteries do. But when Dr. Furchgott applied ACh to strips of rabbit artery, some relaxed while others constricted. Why is that? He soon discovered that the strips that constricted were damaged: Inept laboratory preparation had scraped away or otherwise damaged the artery inner cell lining, the endothelium. No one thought that the endothelium played any sort of role in muscle tone, so lab technicians took no care to preserve it. Dr. Furchgott noted that in intact strips, ACh invariably caused relaxation.

As you will soon see, correcting this oversight propelled the endothelium to the forefront of research on cardiovascular and heart health. This research led to a Nobel Prize for medical research, to the development of Viagra, and, ultimately, to *Great Food, Great Sex*.

Dr. Furchgott did not know what it was about the endothelium that caused relaxation in the presence of ACh. He guessed that the endothelium must produce a mysterious substance that "somehow" does that, and he dubbed it endothelium-derived relaxing factor, or EDRF (Furchgott, 1996). Others noted that this mysterious "somehow" was neither adrenaline nor ACh (both known to impact blood vessels), and so they added the acronym *NANC* (neither adrenaline nor acetylcholine) to *EDRF*.

The noted British scientist Dr. S. Moncada figured out in 1990 that NANC/EDRF is the gas nitric oxide, and that we commonly create it in the body with an enzyme (eNOS) mostly from the amino acid arginine (the L-arginine form)—unlike cattle, which derive it from the nitrogen in their plant food (Moncada and Higgs, 1990). The news that NANC/EDRF is NO initially failed to raise even an eyebrow in many scientific circles. No one believed Dr. Moncada even when he proved that it was NO. In the end, it was Dr. Furchgott (and colleagues) who earned the Nobel Prize in 1998 for the discovery of EDRF.

It was also soon discovered that NO triggers and controls human sexual function, and that the mechanism of human sexual performance is quite dependent on NO. Unlike cattle, we don't graze, so our diet is not exclusively rich in "greens"—nitrogen-rich compounds. We can and do derive NO from the vegetables and legumes in our diet, but we have adapted to meat proteins and so also derive much of our NO from a protein component, the amino acid arginine (Burnett, et al., 1992, 1993, 1995; Rajfer, Aronson, et al., 1992; Wennmalam, Benthin, et al., 1993).

Parenthetically, many amino acids have an L-form and an R-form.

These are mirror-image molecules. The R-form of arginine (R-arginine) is not biologically active in our body; only the L-form is. That is why we dropped the L and refer simply to "arginine."

NERVOUS SYSTEMS

Involuntary body functions such as heartbeat, digestion, and so forth are regulated by the autonomic nervous system (ANS); this is distinct from the peripheral nervous system, which allows us to perceive the world and react to it voluntarily. The ANS consists of two major branches, a sympathetic branch (SNS) that arouses and a parasympathetic branch (PNS) that calms. Ordinarily, there is a dynamic balance between these two branches that keeps order in the body so that neither arousal nor calming prevails unchecked. We call that balance homeostasis. The cardiovascular system is controlled principally by the ANS.

ACTION HORMONES

Your brain and nervous system produce certain hormonal chemical messengers that travel in the bloodstream to targets in the cardiosexual system. Among these are acetylcholine and three others collectively known as catecholamines: adrenaline (epinephrine), noradrenaline (norepinephrine), and dopamine. Catecholamines principally activate the sympathetic branch of the autonomic nervous system.

The pumping action of the heart, its force (stroke volume), and the pulse rate and blood pressure in the arterial blood vessels are controlled by ANS-initiated hormones including the arousing epinephrine and norepinephrine, and the relaxing ACh.

During healthy, normal function, arteries and arterioles are never fully relaxed. The interplay of these hormones keeps them partially constricted. The degree of this partial constriction—called the vasotone—plays a major role in maintaining normal blood pressure at rest. Medical crises where vasotone is lost and blood pressure plummets can be fatal, as we discussed earlier regarding patients using blood-pressure-lowering medications together with PDE5 inhibitors such as Viagra.

Pfizer scientists used this new knowledge of the NANC/EDRF-NO mechanism to further the development of blood-pressure-lowering prescription drugs. They found that in hypertensive individuals, the short-lived effects of NO were even shorter than in people with normal blood pressure. In an attempt to lengthen the duration of NO activity, they developed a compound, a PDE5 inhibitor (Moreland, Goldstein, and Traish, 1998).

As it turned out, the PDE5 inhibitor had only limited usefulness in controlling body blood pressure. The amazing discovery was that men participating in the clinical trials to treat hypertension began to experience penile erections! The erections were due to the fact that PDE5-inhibitor drugs increase the duration of the release of the NO-triggered cGMP, which causes blood vessel dilation in their genitals. And the rest, as they say, is history. Viagra was born, and the sex lives of millions of men and women were changed forever.

WHY *NO* MEANS *YES*

In the normal, healthy state, our action hormones are very sensitive to rapidly changing activity levels. They control the pulse rate and blood circulation appropriate to both increased activity-related metabolism and a calm, relaxed, resting body state. Kidney-related hormones take longer to affect cardiovascular system function.

Until the 1980s, no one knew that there exists another CVS chemical messenger control mechanism that affects both the way that the heart pumps and the way that arterial blood vessels function. That discovery, described on pages 46–47, is the biological role of nitric oxide. It led to a new understanding of endothelium-dependent vasodilation by NO versus that of action hormones (catecholamines) (Furchgott, 1996; Furchgott and Zawadzki, 1990; Moncada and Higgs, 1990).

Briefly, that discovery by Dr. R. Furchgott led to a shift in focus away from the conventional view of blood vessels controlled by ANS-triggered hormones to an "intrinsic" vasodilator substance residing in the endothelium proper. That intrinsic vasodilator substance is cyclic guanosine mono-phosphate (cGMP). Here is how this system works:

- Acetylcholine (ACh) stimulates the endothelium to produce an enzyme, nitric oxide synthase (eNOS).

- eNOS causes the endothelium then to synthesize NO from dietary sources (nitrogen-rich foods, arginine, or other sources).

- NO then causes the release of another enzyme that triggers the endothelium to produce cGMP, causing vessel dilation.

- cGMP is eventually chemically broken down by an enzyme, PDE5, and the constituents are reabsorbed by the body.

- Excess NO is excreted from the body by its conversion to nitrate and nitrite compounds.

This intrinsic relaxation system permits the endothelium to control regional blood flow through the vessels. Viagra and similar compounds are substances that inhibit the action of PDE5 to break down and reabsorb cGMP, thus significantly prolonging the effects of NO on the blood vessels.

NO has an additional curious effect in blood. We have long known that O_2 is taken up by binding with hemoglobin in red blood cells. When O_2 is bound to hemoglobin, it forms oxyhemoglobin. It is in this form that it is transported from the lungs to the organs where O_2 is needed.

We have recently discovered that NO can also bind to hemoglobin, forming nitrosohemoglobin. Nitrosohemoglobin has a special affinity for regions of the body where there is a significant lack of oxygen. When nitrosohemoglobin arrives at one of these locations, it further relaxes the local blood vessels, thereby increasing the regional blood flow and O_2 supply (Jia, Bonaventura, et al., 1996; Stamler, Loh, et al., 1994).

ANTIOXIDANTS: SOLDIERS IN THE BATTLE AGAINST FREE RADICALS

Free radicals are oxygen molecules that have an electrical charge somewhat different from the ordinary form of oxygen on which our life depends. They can do serious damage to our body tissues by interfering with general health—and specifically with sexual function.

Oxygen free radicals can alter the electrical charge of other cells in the body with which they come in contact, changing the way those cells function. The cell membrane is not simply a container that holds the contents of the cell. This membrane is dynamic: Its electrical charge controls the flow of oxygen and nutrients into the cell to support its metabolism, and the flow of carbon dioxide and waste by-products out of the cell. Disturbing the electrical charge of the cells can damage the cell membrane, even kill it.

In the ordinary course of metabolic activity, our body generates free radicals, resulting in what we term oxidative stress. When we are very active, we make more of them than when we are at rest. Fortunately, our body also makes compounds that serve as a mechanism for reducing oxidative stress by eliminating free radicals. One of the most prominent of these is superoxide dismutase (SOD), found in virtually every cell in our body.

Compounds that eliminate free radicals are also called free radical scavengers or antioxidants. Many vitamins such as C and E, minerals such as manganese, and polyphenols like those in vegetables, fruits, and wine are high in antioxidants that serve to "mop up" free radicals.

A new technique, now in use by the US Department of Agriculture (USDA), actually measures the antioxidant capacity of many common foods. That measure is called ORAC, which stands for "oxygen radical absorbance capacity." More about that in chapter 6.

Blood Platelets

Blood has both formed and unformed constituents. Unformed constituents are nutrients, vitamins, minerals, and the like, while others, such as the different cells, have form. Among these are blood platelets. Unlike other cells in blood, such as red blood cells that convey oxygen and carbon dioxide, platelets have no nucleus, and they do not reproduce. Their sole function is to plug up holes due to injury to blood vessels, or to make other repairs to blood vessel walls as the need arises. They do this mostly by forming clots.

Blood platelets usually circulate freely and unchallenged among the other formed and unformed components of blood. But when they are damaged by exposure to free radicals, the electrical charge of their membrane changes; they now tend to clump together in a process medicine calls platelet aggregation.

Platelet aggregation can also damage the membrane of the platelets, causing them to disintegrate and in the process releasing large quantities of serotonin into the bloodstream. The serotonin likewise destabilizes the membranes of other cells in blood by chemically unbalancing their electrical charge and causing the cells to adhere to the endothelium in the lumen (opening) of the vessel.

Blood vessel adhesions interfere with blood flow and have the potential to break off and travel in the bloodstream as clots, causing strokes. This is why many doctors prescribe anticoagulants, also known as blood thinners, to patients at risk for stroke.

Free radicals are hazardous to blood vessels because they can directly damage the endothelium and cause blood pressure to rise. This damage has also been observed to occur in the blood vessels of the penis, and it has been linked directly to erectile dysfunction (Jones, Rees, et al., 2002). This is why the Great Food, Great Sex plan is high in antioxidants.

NO FREE LUNCH

More than 80 percent of Americans have high levels of LDL cholesterol—the bad cholesterol. Some of this percentage is attributable to a genetic propensity for high cholesterol, but for many of us, dietary habits are the main contributor. The fast-food industry has become too adept at squeezing more and more saturated fat into every dish, and fruit and vegetables have only recently penetrated the menu in a form other than ketchup.

The good news is that even a 10 percent decrease in total blood cholesterol levels may reduce the incidence of coronary heart disease by as much as 30 percent. This is why recent medical guidelines encourage more aggressive management of high cholesterol, and why more and more people are being prescribed medications to lower cholesterol. Whether or not you are currently using medication to lower your cholesterol, the Great Food, Great Sex plan is rich in foods that help reduce the hazards of elevated blood cholesterol levels.

Decreased sexual function is like a road sign for the heart that reads DANGER AHEAD. Long before atherosclerosis plagues the cardiovascular system, oxidized LDL cholesterol can be shown to impair sexual function. Oxidized LDL cholesterol actually inhibits the formation of the enzyme needed to synthesize NO in sexual arousal (eNOS). It does this by increasing blood levels of asymmetric dimethylarginine (ADMA), a precursor enzyme (Dai, Zhu, et al., 2004; Li, Zhou, et al., 2004).

Epidemiological studies warn us that elevated serum cholesterol is associated with increased risk of erectile dysfunction, or ED (Schachter, 2000). According to *European Urology,* "Erectile dysfunction is associated with a high prevalence of hyperlipidemia and coronary heart disease" (Roumegerre, Wespes, et al., 2003). Hyperlipidemia means chronically elevated blood cholesterol levels. Elevated blood levels of cholesterol—ordinarily silent and unobservable—are associated with erectile dysfunction, and ED can ". . . serve as a sentinel event for coronary heart disease."

LDL cholesterol in the bloodstream exists as globules, like fat droplets. The problem begins when these globules encounter oxygen free radicals, chemically unstable forms of O_2. Because of their instability, free radicals actively seek an alliance with whatever compound will accept them—and these saturated fats are just the right target.

A simple experiment will illustrate this process: Take a stick of butter and leave it open on the kitchen counter until it becomes rancid. The change in the butter from a delectable, creamy spread to an unappealing curdled pool of fat is an example of free radicals at work. LDL cholesterol globules circulating in the bloodstream can likewise combine with free radicals to form "rancid" oxidized LDL.

Oxidized LDL is identified by macrophages (immune system white blood cells) as foreign matter, and these cells gobble it up. In so doing, they turn themselves into "foam cells." Foam cells seep from the bloodstream into the wall of blood vessels, where they essentially disintegrate, leaving behind debris as well as the oxidized LDL cholesterol. With each successive deposit, a mass forms in the wall, causing injury to the blood vessel walls. Blood platelets are then drawn to the site as part of the vessel wall repair mechanism, and the process of atherosclerosis gets a start.

Blood platelets are drawn to the site of the injury inside the blood vessel wall by way of the blood vessels' very own blood vessels, the vaso vasorum. Blood vessel walls are made up of rings of muscle cells that also need bloodborne O_2. Since the walls are living smooth-muscle-cell rings surrounding an endothelium lining, they have the same O_2, nutrient, and waste elimination requirements as any other tissue in the body. But they cannot communicate directly with the bloodstream, so the vaso vasorum performs that function for them by bringing them blood from the bloodstream and eliminating waste products.

As the mass of macrophage debris and LDL cholesterol sludge accumulates in blood vessel walls, it is plastered over by blood platelets that form a fiber structure, which in turn rapidly accumulates calcium. This mass eventually hardens, forming the basis for atherosclerosis, threatening sexuality and life as well.

The arterial blood vessel wall is composed of three major layers. There is an external layer, the adventitia; next is the media, and then the intima. The endothelium lies on the intima. The vaso vasorum courses through the adventitia, while its branches reach into the intima and also supply the endothelium.

As atherosclerosis forms in the intima of the blood vessel wall, it causes it to bulge into the lumen, thus pushing the endothelium farther and farther from the branches of the vaso vasorum that supply it with oxygen and nutrients and eliminate wastes. The endothelium gradually loses its ability to control the blood vessel by the synthesis of NO. When that happens, the body cannot make enough NO and, thus, cGMP for initiating or sustaining satisfying sexual performance.

By the time the average American is forty-five years old, blood vessel walls may contain nearly half the atherosclerotic plaque that will accumulate in an expected lifetime—and it will only get worse. Since we now know that atherosclerosis interferes directly with sexual vitality, the problem is not due to aging, but with the failure to eat foods that protect the endothelium over the life span.

Women are not exempt from this hazard. In the German journal *Herz* (heart), the authors report that the incidence of female sexual dysfunction (FSD) associated with risk for coronary heart disease is as prevalent as it is in men. The symptoms of FSD are decreased libido, vaginal dryness, pain during intercourse, decreased genital sensation, and orgasmic difficulty (Bernardo, 2001).

HOMOCYSTEINE: BACK IN THE PICTURE

Nearly half the patient population with cardiovascular disease has levels of LDL cholesterol within normal limits. What accounts, then, for their condition?

Dr. Kilmer S. McCully is a researcher whose groundbreaking work in cardiovascular physiology almost forty years ago was dismissed until only recently. As is so often the case, no one believed him when he announced his discovery that the amino acid homocysteine, a by-product of protein metabolism, caused the same kind of damage to arterial blood vessels as LDL cholesterol deposits (McCully, 1969, 1996). He lobbied for years to achieve his well-deserved recognition; now routine doctor office visits often include a test for blood homocysteine levels as part of the blood test panel.

Homocysteine can damage blood vessels. It can be eliminated by a diet rich in vitamins B_{12}, B_6, and folic acid. The three Food Factors in the Great Food, Great Sex plan are high in these nutrients. However, because every individual has a different capacity for absorption, we recommend that you discuss this aspect of your diet with your physician.

HOME OF THE FREE, LAND OF THE HYPERTENSIVE

Americans have a far higher death rate than do people in inland southern Europe, the Mediterranean region, and Japan, even though all these groups have very nearly the same chronically and significantly elevated systolic blood pressure (about 160 mm/Hg).

The incidence of mortality in Americans is about 100 per 10,000. The next highest is 60 per 10,000 for inhabitants of inland southern Europe (France and Spain), then 35 per 10,000 for Mediterranean southern Europeans, and finally 25 per 10,000 for Japanese in Japan (Van den Hoogen, Feskens, et al., 2000).

What could account for these differences? Many authorities reason that for the Europeans, it is the low-animal-fat Mediterranean diet, which consists principally of nitrate-rich fresh vegetables and antioxidant-rich fresh fruits, olive products, and wines (Trichopoulou and Critselis, 2004;

Trichopoulou and Vasilopoulou, 2000). The Japanese diet is also high in fresh fruits and vegetables and, in coastal areas and Okinawa, in fish as well (Sauvaget, Nagano, et al., 2003).

The Ankle-Brachial Index

There is a simple measure by which you can gain insight into the status of your circulatory system. Called the Ankle-Brachial Index (ABI), it is the ratio of blood pressure measured at your ankle to blood pressure measured at your arm. The ABI estimates the extent of atherosclerotic plaque deposition in your arterial blood vessels (Hooi, Kester, et al., 2004; Murabito, Evans, et al., 2003). You may wish to ask your physician to perform this simple test during your next office visit.

We also believe that the difference in the incidence of death from coronary heart disease between Americans and other cultural groups is due to diet. Specifically, there is a demonstrably protective effect with higher consumption of our *three Food Factors for sexual vitality*. Most importantly, researchers agree that protection of the endothelium confers distinct benefit (Fuentes, Lopez-Miranda, et al., 2002; Leighton, Cuevas, et al., 1999).

The National Heart, Lung, and Blood Institute (NHLBI) has begun to lead the charge by guiding consumers to nitrogen-rich foods to lower blood pressure and protect the cardiovascular system and the heart. Ongoing clinical trials continue to look at the impact of diet on cardiovascular disease. As long ago as 1996, the American Heart Association (AHA) sponsored clinical trials to show that oral supplementation of arginine boosts heart health (Rector, Bank, et al., 1996; Blum and Miller, 1999). Our food plan incorporates the latest thinking in cardiovascular nutrition and gives you a great reason to stay on our diet—better and more enjoyable sex.

ESTROGEN AND THE ENDOTHELIUM IN WOMEN

Estrogen promotes healthy function of the endothelium in women and helps protect them against the formation of atherosclerosis. In fact, the lower incidence of hypertension and coronary artery disease in pre-menopausal women compared with men versus the higher incidence in postmenopausal women has been shown to be related to the protective effects of estrogen on the endothelium (Orshal and Khalil, 2004).

Decreasing estrogen production as women approach menopause causes an increase in ADMA, a substance that inhibits the release of the enzyme eNOS necessary to the formation of NO. This biological phenomenon puts women at increased risk for cardiovascular and heart disease at the same time that it jeopardizes sexual function and vitality (Li, Zhou, et al., 2004). Despite recent concerns about estrogen replacement therapy (ERT), it has been shown to lower plasma levels of ADMA in healthy postmenopausal women.

Although estrogen confers some degree of protection of the endothelium in women by reducing ADMA, inhibiting the oxidation of LDL cholesterol also reduces ADMA. In fact, postmenopausal women are even more susceptible to the damaging effects of oxidized LDL cholesterol because they do not have the protection afforded by estrogen in pre- and perimenopausal women (Wakatsuki, Ikenoue, et al., 2004). As we have discussed earlier, the Great Food, Great Sex plan is designed to counteract these effects through a high level of antioxidants found in particular foods.

EVERY CLOUD HAS A SILVER (ENDOTHELIAL) LINING

The key to success in the bedroom for the rest of your life is maintaining the health of the endothelial lining of the arterial blood vessels all through your body. Healthy endothelium function will be able to produce that all-important NO when you want it and where you need it.

Optimal cardiosexual function is provided by the endothelium. Love-making differs from other cardiovascular functions in your body only in anatomical "geography." And in this case, an ounce of prevention is definitely worth a pound of cure.

Join us now for a delicious dietary excursion that should take you from the kitchen to the bedroom, as you learn all about the three Food Factors of our Great Food, Great Sex plan.

4

Factor 1 Foods—Greens and Beans

Nitrogen-Rich Foods

If your idea of a green vegetable is the pickle served with your pastrami sandwich, or the olive in your martini, please read this chapter carefully. Sexual vitality depends on the readiness of the endothelium to deliver nitric oxide (NO) to the sex organs when aroused in order to produce erection in men, and vaginal and clitoral engorgement and lubrication in women.

The endothelium forms NO from two major dietary sources:

- Factor 1 Foods, such as vegetables and legumes—a fancy term for beans.

- Factor 2 Foods—rich sources of the amino acid arginine, which are described in the next chapter.

Factor 1 Foods, green vegetables and legumes, can deliver NO from natural nitrogen compounds and amino acids, nitrates (NO_2), and, in some cases, nitrites (NO_3).

The body will dramatically increase NO production in response to a number of challenging conditions, including vigorous exercise, sexual arousal, and even inflammatory immune response. But nitric oxide has a very short life in the body, and it must be made continuously to meet these challenges. A few seconds after NO is produced, it is eliminated by the body in urine as nitrate (NO_2) and nitrite (NO_3).

When the body raises NO production, both blood serum and urinary excretion of these two compounds rise accordingly. Thus, nitrate and nitrite serum levels and excretion in urine are reliable markers of NO production (Wennmalam, Benthin, et al., 1993).

TYPICAL AMERICAN DIET = TYPICAL AMERICAN SEX LIFE

Highly desirable NO production results primarily from the foods we eat on a daily basis. And while it is true that meat and potatoes contain substantial amounts of arginine, the typical American diet of high-fat red meat and french fries has a devastating impact on the endothelium of our arterial blood vessels. The nitric oxide needed both for cardiovascular health and sexual vitality requires healthy vessels for production as well as transport. Cholesterol directly impairs NO production and, in both the short and long run, impairs sexual vitality.

When there is damage to the endothelium from hypertension, heart disease, or chronic elevated serum LDL cholesterol, NO production is lowered by that damage; serum levels and urinary excretion of nitrate and nitrite are also lower than expected (Golikov and Nikolaeva, 2004). A report in the *Journal of Cardiovascular Pharmacology* confirmed that patients with hypertension also have lower-than-normal urinary excretion of nitrate and nitrite (Surdacki, Nowicki, et al., 1999). The journal *Hypertension* has also reported that patients with essential (chronic) hypertension have a lower level of NO availability, which is reflected in lower-than-normal serum levels of nitrate and nitrite (Node, Kitakaze, et al., 1997).

If left elevated, serum cholesterol will damage the blood vessels, the cardiovascular system, and the heart permanently, resulting in vasculo-genic (originating in blood vessels) sexual dysfunction, which is extremely resistant to treatment (Siroky and Azadzoi, 2003). Elevated serum cholesterol not only increases the risk of heart disease but is also known to be a direct risk factor for erectile dysfunction (ED) in men.

In a recent study, ED was treated successfully by lowering serum cholesterol with medication (Saltzman, Guay, et al., 2004). The authors reported that "Erectile function improves in men with hypercholesterolemia [chronic elevated blood cholesterol levels] as the only risk factor for ED when treated with atorvastatin."

The good news is that it is well established that, except for individuals with a genetic form of severe hypercholesterolemia, cholesterol levels can be directly and positively improved by dietary change. According to researchers at the University of South Carolina, men with lower blood LDL cholesterol or higher blood HDL cholesterol may be less likely to develop erectile dysfunction (www.people.virginia.edu/~rjh9u/impotent.html).

Numerous phytochemical (plant-derived) constituents in vegetables and legumes confer protection from cholesterol oxidation, and increasing your consumption of these foods can also provide both major short- and long-term benefits. The *Journal of the American College of Cardiology* reported in 2003 that, amazingly, adding a green salad to a high-fat meal can reduce the immediate adverse impact of the ingested fat as well as promoting NO production in the body (Plotnick, Corretti, et al., 2003). Another good reason to make a large salad your first course—a delicious form of nutrition-packed foreplay.

THE NIH HIGH-NITROGEN-COMPOUND CLINICAL TRIALS

As we have seen, cardiovascular health *and* sexual vitality depend on the ready availability of nitric oxide, derived from the endothelium. Above the waist, cardiovascular health depends on the ability of NO to maintain adequate blood circulation and normal blood pressure throughout the body, and to protect the endothelium (on which NO production depends) from free radicals and oxidized LDL cholesterol. Sexual vitality is maintained and nourished through the same circulatory system below the waist as well.

The heart is the only pump for blood that serves the body. Blood pressure rises and falls with muscle activity level in all parts of the body except the brain, where it remains more or less constant. Rising and falling with metabolic demands, blood pressure is more or less the same in the major blood vessels coursing through the body, including the blood vessels that lead to the erectile chambers of the penis.

Yet in the flaccid penis, the arteries are constantly somewhat constricted; blood is not flowing through them at the same rate as it is flowing elsewhere in the body. Erection and extension result from *relaxation* of the blood vessels in the penis, relaxation that allows increased blood inflow into that organ. Contrary to common myth, it is not due to muscle contraction.

It seems counterintuitive: Why isn't the blood pressure in the penis the same as it is throughout the body? Why isn't the penis erect all the time? After all, there is no separate blood pump for the penis.

The answer is that the blood vessels in the penis are uniquely controlled by a special mechanism that keeps them always partially constricted (narrowed). But we now understand that in sexual arousal and erection, the blood vessels are commanded to relax, allowing body blood pressure to fill the spongy erectile chambers of the penis. As the penis fills and expands, the expansion constricts the veins that would convey blood out, and so blood pressure in the penis rises higher than body blood pressure, and it is maintained so long as the biochemical message that causes the blood vessels to relax is still in effect.

Sexual response in women, namely the mechanism of vaginal and clitoral engorgement and lubrication, depends on the same biochemical message to relax blood vessels and increase blood flow to the sex organs (Burnett, Calvin, et al., 1997; D'Amati, di Gioia, et al., 2002; Moreland, Goldstein, and Traish, 1998; Park, Moreland, et al., 1998).

This relationship of NO-producing foods with cardiovascular health resulted in a large-scale nutritional study currently under way sponsored by the National Heart, Lung, and Blood Institute (NHLBI) of the National Institutes of Health (NIH). The study is designed to raise NO availability through a high-nitrogen-compound diet. We have included a number of the recipes developed for this trial in our six-week plan. (To learn more about access to clinical trials, visit www.clinicaltrials.gov/ct/gui/show/NCT00069654.)

Arousal depends on the very same NO mechanism that ensures cardiovascular health. Factor 1 Foods, Greens and Beans, provide a ready dietary stream of NO production, critical to successful lovemaking for women and men. (One hopes that the government will eventually monitor sexual function as one of its quality-of-life measures—it might make trial recruitment easier.) A food plan that includes adequate quantities of greens and beans provides the body with the necessary ingredients to produce lots of NO. These foods have also been shown to actually reverse endothelium damage and thus increase NO availability.

"I'M STRONG TO THE FINISH 'CAUSE I EATS ME SPINACH"

Popeye was correct in attributing his energy to a deep green food. Factor 1 Foods contribute to sexual vitality in these principal ways:

- First, they are a ready supply of plant-derived nitrogen compounds from which the body can derive nitric oxide.

- Second, they provide numerous phytochemical constituents— primarily in the form of biologically active pigments—that directly lower serum cholesterol, especially saponin in legumes (beans), and phthalides (Francis, Kerem, et al., 2002).

This food group is also rich in folate (folic acid), vitamins B_6 and B_{12}, vitamins E and C, flavonoids, and phytoestrogens, which help to lower both serum cholesterol and homocysteine, and thus protect the cardiovascular system (Tucker, 2004).

These foods are easy to identify by either their deep green color or, in the case of beans, their shape. How can you tell how rich your diet is in nitrogen compounds? Short of laboratory analysis (commonly the Kjeldahl technique), most sources take crude protein as the best estimate of nitrogen content. Below we list common foods in the Great Food, Great Sex plan's Greens and Beans category. This is a short list of the sexiest players of this group.

COMMON FACTOR 1 FOODS

Arginine values (see chapter 5), where known, are provided along with other nutritional information for each item below.

Artichokes

A single artichoke is actually an unopened flower bud. Related to the thistle family, *Cynara scolymus* is a green cone-shaped bud consisting of several parts: overlapping spiny-tipped tough outer leaves with a tender fleshy base and an inedible choke, or thistle, which is enclosed within a light-colored cone of immature leaves; and a round, firm-fleshed base. This meaty base, technically called the bottom, is the jewel within the crown of thorns. Commercially available artichoke "hearts" come from tiny whole artichokes. The artichoke is also a rich source of vitamin C, folate, dietary fiber, and a multitude of minerals.

- *1 large artichoke: 5 g protein, 76 calories, 0.2 g total fat, 152 mg sodium.*

Asparagus

Asparagus contains an impressive supply of folic acid as well as some vitamin C and, in green asparagus, some beta-carotene. Asparagus also contains the phytochemical glutathione, a powerful antioxidant.

- *1-cup serving, cooked: 5 g protein, 143 mg arginine, 43 calories, 0.6 g total fat, 20 mg sodium.*

Beans

Dried beans are a dietary staple in many cultures because they offer an abundant supply of complex (slowly digested) carbohydrates as well as protein. In fact, beans contain a higher proportion of protein than any other plant food. Because the protein is incomplete (missing some essential amino acids) bean dishes should be complemented with rice, other grains, or nuts (or, for nonvegetarians, a small amount of animal protein, such as chicken, fish, cheese, or yogurt) to supply the missing amino acids.

After soaking beans, pour off the soaking water, then add the required amount of fresh water or broth; the liquid should cover the beans by about 2 inches. Bring the liquid slowly to a boil, skimming off the scum that rises to the surface. When the liquid boils, reduce the heat, partially cover the pot, and simmer until the beans are tender. Stir occasionally, adding more water if necessary. The beans are done when they can be easily pierced with the tip of a knife.

The amount of time it takes to cook beans varies with the size, density, and age of the beans. Small beans such as mung and adzuki take 30 to 40 minutes (after soaking). Medium-sized beans (the bulk of the bean family), such as black beans and kidney beans, take 1 hour to 1 hour and 20 minutes.

Cooked beans can be frozen in plastic bags, so don't hesitate to make a pound at a time. Precooked beans can help make a meal in a minute with the sexy chef's touch in it.

Pinto Beans

These medium-sized long "painted" beans are a reddish tan, mottled with brown flecks. The most popular beans in the United States, they contain more fiber than any other legume. Their earthy flavor makes them a favorite in Mexican dishes; they can be substituted for kidney beans in chili.

- *1-cup serving, cooked: 41 g protein, 2,115 mg arginine, 670 calories, 1 g total fat, 23 mg sodium.*

Red Beans

These are medium-sized oval beans with a terra-cotta color, and they have a rich, savory flavor that makes them the perfect choice for chilies or soups, or for combining with rice.

- *1-cup serving, raw: 41 g protein, 2,567 mg arginine, 620 calories, 29 g total fat, 22 mg sodium.*

Lima Beans

Lima beans come in two sizes: large limas, called Fordhooks or butter beans, and baby limas, a smaller, milder-tasting variety. Both are sold frozen as well as dried and canned.

- *1-cup serving, cooked: 38 g protein, 2,594 mg arginine, 602 calories, 1 g total fat, 32 mg sodium.*

White Beans

Delicious in soups and stews, these beans are hearty yet mild-flavored.

- *1-cup serving, cooked: 41 g protein, 2,115 mg arginine, 673 calories, 0.2 g total fat, 23 mg sodium.*

Black Beans

These beans are pea-sized and have a somewhat smoky flavor. They are a common ingredient in many Latin American dishes, including black beans and rice, refried beans, bean burritos, and black bean soup. They are also used in Chinese black bean sauce.

- *1-cup serving, cooked: 42 g protein, 2,594 mg arginine, 662 calories, 2.75 g total fat, 10 mg sodium.*

Kidney Beans

These beans, named for their shape, may be dark red, light red, or white. They are the main ingredient in chili, and like all beans can be added to soups, salads, and casseroles. White kidney beans are known as cannellini, and are the beans commonly found in Italian dishes such as minestrone soup.

- *1-cup serving, cooked: 45 g protein, 2,777 mg arginine, 607 calories, 0.5 g total fat, 20 mg sodium.*

Chickpeas

Chickpeas, or garbanzos, are a good source of low-fat, high-protein, and complex carbohydrates; fiber (including the soluble fiber that may lower cholesterol); and B vitamins—especially folate and minerals.

Chickpeas, probably originating in the Middle East, are a common feature in many cuisines, ranging from Middle Eastern to Indian, Italian, Spanish, and Latin American. Chickpeas are extremely versatile, and their delicate nutlike flavor makes them an excellent addition to many recipes, including salads, soups, dips, and pasta or grain dishes. When roasted, chickpeas resemble nuts and make a tasty snack. Falafel is a popular Middle Eastern dish in which the mashed beans are formed into balls and deep-fried.

- *1-cup serving, cooked: 38.6 g protein, 3,638 mg arginine, 728 calories, 12 g total fat, 48 mg sodium.*

Bok Choy

Bok choy, also known as pak choi or Peking cabbage, has plump white stalks and deep green leaves. Similar to other cabbages, it is rich in vitamin C and contains significant amounts of nitrogen compounds known as indoles, as well as fiber. It is also a good source of folic acid. Its deep green leaves have more beta-carotene than other cabbages, and it also supplies considerably more calcium. It is a common vegetable in Asian dishes, and a great way to add volume to a dish without a load of calories.

- *1-cup serving, cooked: 3 g protein, 20 calories, 0.3 g total fat, 58 mg sodium.*

Broccoli

Broccoli packs a powerful nutritional punch. Rich in vitamins and minerals, notably vitamin C, folate (folic acid), and potassium, this deep green food also contains a considerable amount of beta-carotene. Broccoli, like all green vegetables, is low in calories and virtually fat-free.

- *1-cup serving, raw: 5 g protein, 168 mg arginine, 44 calories, 0.5 g total fat, 41 mg sodium.*

Brussels Sprouts

Brussels sprouts look like little heads of cabbage—not surprising, since both belong to the same botanical family. Some markets offer brussels sprouts on the stalk, but often the sprouts are cut off before going to market.

Brussels sprouts have a slightly milder flavor and denser texture than their cabbage cousins. They contain the nitrogen compounds, indoles, and a significant amount of vitamin C. Brussels sprouts also supply folic acid, potassium, vitamin K, and a small amount of beta-carotene.

- *1-cup serving, raw: 3 g protein, 179 mg arginine, 38 calories, zero fat, 22 mg sodium.*

Cabbage, Green

Cabbage is a member of the large family of cruciferous vegetables (see below). It contains significant amounts of nitrogen compounds, indoles, and fiber, both soluble and insoluble, as well as vitamin C. Cabbage can be grated raw for coleslaw or cooked in a wide variety of recipes.

- *1-cup serving, cooked: 1 g protein, 18 calories, 0.3 g total fat, 13 mg sodium.*

Cauliflower

Cauliflower—like its closest relative, broccoli—is a cruciferous vegetable. *Cruciferous* is derived from the word *cross*. These plants have four petals arranged like the arms and trunk of a cross. The cruciferous vegetables include radishes and turnips. While broccoli opens outward to sprout bunches of green florets, cauliflower forms a compact head of undeveloped white flower buds. Cauliflower grows on a single stalk, and the head of the plant is surrounded by heavily ribbed green leaves that protect it from sunlight. The flower buds never develop chlorophyll, and thus remain white.

Some markets sell a cauliflower-broccoli hybrid that looks like cauliflower but has a green curd. Less dense than the white kind, this recently developed variety cooks more quickly and has a milder taste.

- *1-cup florets, cooked: 2 g protein, 95 mg arginine, 29 calories, 0.6 g total fat, 19 mg sodium.*

Celery

Celery is generally enjoyed raw, as an appetizer or salad ingredient, but is also a flavorful addition to many cooked dishes. A bunch or head of celery is made up of individual stalks or ribs. These ribs are naturally crisp due to the rigidity of the plant's cell walls and the high water content within the cells. Because celery is mostly water, it is exceptionally low in calories and makes a crispy, satisfying snack food with very few calories (just don't dip it in creamy dressing). Celery provides potassium, but is relatively low in other nutrients. The tops of the celery are somewhat bitter if eaten raw, but are wonderful in soup stock and stews.

- *1-cup serving, chopped: 0.9 g protein, 22 mg arginine, 19 calories, 0.2 g total fat, 104 mg sodium.*

Collard Greens

Enjoyed as a side dish in Southern cuisine, deep green collards are a good source of vitamin C and are rich in phytochemicals, including sulforaphane and indoles. Levels of beta-carotene and other nutrients in leafy greens appear to be linked to the presence of chlorophyll, the green pigment produced by photosynthesis. So the deep color of these greens signals that collards (unlike their paler cabbage-family cousins) are also rich in beta-carotene.

Collards are a good source of folate and B vitamins; they also supply a substantial amount of calcium. Their large, smooth leaves, which are deep green in color, don't form a head, but grow outward from a central axis.

Each leaf is attached to a long, heavy stalk (which is inedible). Collards are one of the milder greens, with a pleasantly bitter flavor somewhere between cabbage and kale.

- *1-cup serving: 4 g protein, 45 mg arginine, 49 calories, 0.7 g total fat, 17 mg sodium.*

Cucumbers

The cucumber belongs to the same vegetable family as pumpkin, zucchini (a close lookalike), watermelon, and other squashes. First cultivated in Asia in ancient times, it was brought to America by Columbus, and was eventually grown by both Native Americans and colonists from Florida to Canada. Like celery, cucumbers have a very high water content, giving them a crisp, cool taste.

There are two basic types of cucumbers, slicing varieties that are eaten fresh, and those cultivated for pickling. The slicing cucumbers sold in most supermarkets are field-grown varieties that are usually 6 to 9 inches long and have glossy, dark green skin and tapering ends. After harvesting, the skin is often waxed for longer shelf life, so peeling is advised.

More recently, greenhouse slicing cucumbers have come on the market. Sometimes called European or English cucumbers, they are thinner, ridged, and 1 to 2 feet in length. The majority are also seedless, milder-flavored, and, for many people, easier to digest ("burpless"). Pickling varieties are smaller and squatter, and have bumpy, light green skins. One type, the kirby, which is used to make commercial dill pickles, is also sold fresh (and usually unwaxed). Cucumber lovers appreciate fresh kirbies for their thin skin, crisp flesh, and tiny seeds.

- *1 medium cucumber: 1 g protein, 22.5 mg arginine, 24 calories, 0.3 g total fat, 4 mg sodium.*

Jerusalem Artichoke

Despite its name, the Jerusalem artichoke is not an artichoke—nor does it originate in Jerusalem. It is alternately called sunchoke. The sunchoke is a tuber, or underground stem, that resembles a small knobby potato or a piece of gingerroot. Loved for its sweet, nutty taste and crisp texture, it can be eaten raw or cooked and added to all types of dishes. It is almost as rich in iron as meats but has no fat.

In order to preserve the nutrients in their skin, scrub sunchokes well with a vegetable brush rather than peeling them. To prevent discoloration, put sliced sunchokes in cold water with some lemon juice or vinegar. When sunchokes are cooked unpeeled, they will darken because of their iron content.

- *6 ounces: 3 g protein, 114 calories, zero total fat and cholesterol, 6 mg sodium.*

Kale

Kale is another member of the cabbage family, and is a good source of vitamin C, sulforaphane, and indoles. Kale has a substantial mineral content, providing manganese as well as some iron, calcium, and potassium. There is also antioxidant vitamin E in the flavorful leaves.

Kale is similar to collards, except that its leaves are curly at the edges. It has a stronger flavor and a coarser texture. The most common variety is deep green, but others are yellow-green, red, or purple, with either plain flat or ruffled leaves. The colored varieties, sometimes called salad savoy, are most often grown for ornamental purposes, but they are edible. However, they do have a stronger flavor than regular kale.

- *1-cup serving, chopped, raw: 2 g protein, 123 mg arginine, 33 calories, zero total fat, 29 mg sodium.*

Lettuce

Every American now consumes about 30 pounds of lettuce a year, five times more than they ate a hundred years ago. Due to improved methods of shipping and storage, salad greens are some of the most widely available fresh vegetables on the market. Iceberg lettuce is the most popular, but also the least nutritious, member of the lettuce family. As we grow more adventurous, we are adding a wider variety of greens to our salad bowls, such as mesclun and romaine.

In general, the darker green the leaves, the more nutritious the salad green. For example, romaine and watercress have seven to eight times as much beta-carotene, two to four times the calcium, and twice the potassium of iceberg lettuce. By varying the greens in your salads, you can enhance the nutritional content as well as varying tastes and textures.

- *55-g serving, raw: 1 g protein, 38.5 mg arginine, 7 calories, zero total fat, 3 mg sodium.*

Peas

Green garden peas are legumes, plants that produce pods enclosing fleshy seeds. Dried beans such as chickpeas, split peas, and the others described on pages 64–65 require long cooking times, but green peas are packaged and prepared like all fresh green vegetables. Green peas are second only to lima beans as a fresh vegetable source of protein: 1 cup of peas contains more protein than a whole egg, or a tablespoon of peanut butter, yet it has less than half a gram of fat.

Frozen green peas retain their color, flavor, and nutrients better than canned peas and are much lower in sodium. If thawed and not cooked, frozen peas can be substituted for fresh peas in salads and other uncooked dishes.

Fresh snow peas and sugar snap peas are now more readily available. These peas have an edible pod and are meant to be eaten cooked or raw, with the pod intact. Snow peas—also called sugar peas and Chinese pea pods—have pale green, flat pods with small, immature-looking peas because they are picked before the seeds have developed in the pod. Sugar snaps were created in the 1970s as a cross between the snow pea and green pea. They have plump edible pods filled with extremely sweet and tender peas.

- *1-cup serving, raw: 8 g protein, 621 mg arginine, 117 calories, 1 g total fat, 7 mg sodium.*

Potatoes

Potatoes contain an energizing supply of complex carbohydrates plus protein and important vitamins and minerals, including potassium, vitamins B_6 and C, copper, and manganese.

Americans on average consume about 126 pounds of potatoes per person per year—far more than any other vegetable, and much of it in the form of fat-laden chips and french fries. That comes to about 35 billion pounds of potatoes annually. In fact, simply by virtue of the quantities eaten, the potato is the leading source of vitamin C in the American diet.

There are many varieties of potatoes that can accommodate many different dishes. Smaller potatoes like round reds (sometimes called new potatoes) are good for boiling or adding to soups. They have a high moisture and sugar content so they cook quickly and have a delicately sweet flavor. Larger potatoes such as russets (sometimes called Idaho potatoes) have a starchier texture and are delicious baked or mashed.

- *1 medium potato, raw: 3 g protein, 132 mg arginine, 144 calories, zero total fat, 4 mg sodium.*

Spinach

Spinach is a rich source of carotenoids, including beta-carotene and lutein, and also contains quercetin, a phytochemical with antioxidant properties. It's high in vitamins and minerals, particularly folate, vitamin K, magnesium, and manganese. It also contains more protein than most vegetables, although the protein is incomplete—spinach and other leafy green vegetables are low in the amino acid methionine.

Raw spinach is a healthy addition to salads, but in order to get the full benefits of absorbable carotenoid antioxidants, it is best cooked. Fresh spinach must be thoroughly rinsed before eating to wash away sand and grit that cling to the leaves.

Savoy spinach has crinkly, curly leaves with a dark green color. It is the type sold in fresh bunches at most markets. Springy and crisp, it's particularly good in salads. The flat or smooth-leaf spinach has unwrinkled spade-shaped leaves that are easier to clean than the savoy. This type is generally used for canned and frozen spinach as well as soups, baby foods, and other processed foods. The semi-savoy, increasingly popular, has slightly crinkled leaves offering some of the texture of savoy, but is not as difficult to clean.

- *1-cup serving, raw: 1 g protein, 48.6 mg arginine, 7 calories, zero total fat, 24 mg sodium.*

Sprouts

The most common are the alfalfa seed and mung bean sprouts. In growing from seed to sprout, there is a loss of nutritional value because most of the carbohydrate and fat in the seed is used for growth. On the plus side, sprouts hold some B vitamins and iron, and can serve as a filling, high-water-content, low-calorie food. Sprouts are a great way to stretch a sandwich or a salad without piling on calories.

Alfalfa Sprouts

These delicate white sprouts with green tops have a mild, nutty flavor.

- *1-cup serving: 4 g protein, 10 calories, zero fat and cholesterol, 2 mg sodium.*

Mung Bean Sprouts

The most typical bean sprouts, much thicker than alfafa, these white sprouts are often found in Asian dishes and are excellent in stir-fries, soups, and salads.

- *1-cup serving: 3 g protein, 31 calories, 0.2 g total fat, zero cholesterol, 6 mg sodium.*

String Beans

Fresh string beans offer some vitamin C, folate, iron, and, if they're deep green in color, some beta-carotene.

String or snap beans are the most popular fresh beans. The "string" that runs along the seam of the bean has been bred out of most modern varieties. These beans are actually immature kidney beans, and their pods can be flat, oval, or rounded. The most familiar types are green beans and yellow wax beans, which are identical in taste and texture (yellow beans, however, contain less beta-carotene).

Italian green beans, also called Romano beans, are distinguished by broad, flat, bright green pods. They are most often available in frozen form but can also be found fresh in local farmers' markets and specialty stores. Purple wax beans, similar to small yellow wax beans, have a dark purple pod that turns green when cooked. Scarlet runner beans have broad pods; they're flat and green. The seeds (beans) are scarlet.

- *1-cup serving, raw: 2 g protein, 80.3 mg arginine, 44 calories, zero total fat, 4 mg sodium.*

Swiss Chard

Swiss chard, also known simply as chard, comes from a variety of beets grown specifically for their stems and leaves. Swiss chard has a milder flavor than other cooking greens and its dark green leaves are wider and flatter than beet greens. The fleshy stalks and ribs are either white or, as in red (ruby) chard, a jewel-like red. Unlike many greens, the stalks of Swiss chard are completely edible. In fact, in European countries they are considered the best part of the plant. Unless the chard is young, the stalks should be separated from the leaves and given a little extra cooking time.

- *1-cup serving, raw: 1 g protein, 42.1 mg arginine, 7 calories, zero total fat, 77 mg sodium.*

Turnips

Turnips are related to cabbage and are a good source of complex carbohydrates. Their greens are also edible and are rich in vitamins and minerals. Turnips come in an astonishing range of shapes and sizes, depending on the age and variety: Some are the size of golf balls, while others can reach as much as 40 to 50 pounds. The flesh can be white or yellow, but most commercial turnips have white flesh.

- *1-cup serving, cooked/boiled: 1 g protein, 29.6 mg arginine, 34 calories, zero total fat, 25 mg sodium.*

Factor 2 Foods—Staminators

Power Up Your Love Life

As you may have guessed from the title of this chapter, Factor 2 Foods are the power lifters of sexual vitality. These protein building blocks provide the highest values of arginine, the amino acid that is one of the body's principal sources of the gas nitric oxide (NO). NO, it turns out, is just as biologically active as are the gases oxygen (O_2) and carbon dioxide (CO_2).

The body derives NO from two major dietary sources: the amino acid arginine, found in meats, nuts, dairy products, and vegetable proteins, and the nitrogen compounds in green vegetables and legumes (Food Factor 1, Greens and Beans).

ARGININE

Arginine* not only helps directly with physiological sexual function but, as previously noted, also provides proven medical benefits to patients with hypertension, elevated serum cholesterol, heart disease, and diabetes—all of which jeopardize sexual vitality.

*Since only the L-form of arginine (L-arginine) is biologically active, we uniformly refer here to it as "arginine."

Arginine and NO are hot topics in science today because of their relationship to cardiovascular function and health. The Library of the National Academy of Sciences cites 61,260 medical publications keyworded to "arginine, cardiovascular." There are 19,480 keyed to "nitric oxide, cardiovascular" as of January 2005. These can be found in prestigious medical journals such as the *American Journal of Hypertension, Annals of Internal Medicine, Cardiology, Circulation, Hypertension, The Lancet,* the *Journal of the American College of Cardiology, Proceedings of the National Academy of Sciences (USA),* the *Journal of Clinical Investigation,* the *Journal of the American Medical Association,* and *New England Journal of Medicine,* to mention just a few.

What is not receiving adequate attention are the links among arginine, NO, and sexuality.

We now know that there are at least three forms of the enzyme nitric oxide synthase (NOS) linked to three different physiological systems in the body:

- The greatest quantity of NO is produced by NOS in immune system cells such as macrophages and lymphocytes, and it is used by them to destroy foreign invaders like bacteria, parasites, molds, fungi, viruses, and internal "invaders" such as cancer cells. To that end, in the stomach they take up almost half of the dietary arginine consumed in the diet (Bistrian, 2004).

- The nerves and brain have their own form of NOS. They use NO in their communication function and, we believe, in data storage in the brain (Kiss, Zsilla, and Vizi, 2004).

- The cardiovascular system (CVS) provides the infrastructure for sexual vitality. The CVS gets its NO from a form of NOS in the endothelium lining of arterial blood vessels. That is why we refer to it as eNOS. Nitric oxide in the cardiovascular system serves to control blood flow in the circulatory system and also modulate the action of the heart. However, NO engages in two other major CVS protective functions: It is an antioxidant that can eliminate oxygen free radicals, and it can also lower serum low-density lipoprotein (LDL) cholesterol—even reduce and eliminate atherosclerotic plaque that causes the potentially deadly hardening of the arteries.

Research has shown that NO is essential to health and that arginine is probably the chief raw material the body uses to make it. It is also clear that increasing arginine availability through diet is also beneficial. Medical research suggests that the typical American diet is deficient in arginine, which has dire health consequences for all the functions dependent on NO production, especially immune function, cardiovascular and heart function, and sexual function.

We all accept that nutritional deficiencies can produce illness. This was shown definitively as early as the mid-1700s by Dr. James Lind, a British naval surgeon who proved that consumption of citrus fruits could prolong the life of sailors suffering from scurvy. Many years later, Nobel Prize–winning research by Dr. Albert Szent-Gyorgyi refined this hypothesis by showing that what Lind was "supplementing" was ascorbic acid, or vitamin C.

Because of our high national incidence of elevated blood pressure and cholesterol, we hypothesize that many Americans may be suffering from an arginine deficiency. This is supported by research on the success of treatment with oral arginine supplementation for patients with various medical conditions:

• **Hypertension.** The journal of the American Heart Association (AHA), *Circulation*, reported that patients with untreated hypertension were given 2 g arginine per day for one week. At the end of that period, their blood pressure was significantly reduced. No changes were noted in a comparable control group (Pagnotta, Germano, et al., 1997).

• **Heart function.** The same journal also reported that patients with heart failure given 5.6 to 12.6 g oral arginine per day for six weeks showed significant improvement in ability to exercise and other functions (Rector, Bank, et al., 1996).

• **Elevated serum cholesterol and atherosclerosis.** The *International Journal of Cardiovascular Interventions* reported that arginine reduces platelet aggregation and improves blood circulation in men with coronary artery disease and atherosclerosis (Blum and Miller, 1999). In young adults who do not yet have noticeable evidence of atherosclerosis, elevated serum LDL cholesterol may result in the inability of the endothelium to signal blood vessels to dilate to increase regional blood flow. The *Journal of Clinical Investigation* reported that oral arginine supplementation significantly improved blood circulation (Clarkson, Adams, et al., 1996).

• **Diabetes.** *Diabetes Care* has reported that long-term administration of oral arginine improves peripheral and hepatic insulin sensitivity in type 2 diabetes (Piatti, Monti, et al., 2001).

And finally, regarding sexual function:

• **Erectile function.** The *International Journal of Impotence Research* reported in 1994 that oral arginine taken for two weeks significantly improved erectile function in impotent men, as compared with controls. The *Journal of Sex and Marital Therapy* has reported a study in which arginine was given in combination with pycnogenol (see page 116). The combination dramatically increased the effectiveness of arginine, and restored sexual function to a significant number of previously impotent men (Stanislavov and Nikolova, 2003).

These seemingly different medical conditions all have in common a negative impact on cardiovascular function that poses a direct threat to sexual vitality. The Staminators are foods rich in arginine that enhance sexual vitality by supplying ample NO.

DIETARY ARGININE: YOUR FRONT-LINE DEFENSE

When you consume arginine in foods or supplements, only some of it becomes available to the endothelium for forming NO. Some amino acids such as lysine can interfere with its absorption, and certain specialized immune cells (macrophages) in the gut gobble up a lot of it—further reducing the amount that enters the bloodstream. All in all, only about half of the arginine you ingest in food or supplements actually makes it to your circulatory system.

Long before nutritionists learned how to mass-produce arginine for use in supplements, the only way to get sufficient amounts of it was to eat food products rich in it. The twenty-two amino acids that we require to stay alive are plentiful in meat, poultry, fish, eggs, and dairy products. Wild game is particularly high in arginine. There are more than 5 g in a single pound of venison or buffalo meat.

Arginine can also be found in certain vegetable sources—particularly wheat germ, legumes, nuts, and seeds. Nuts, in particular, are very high in arginine. Fruits and vegetables, jam-packed as they are with other vital nutrients, contain almost no arginine.

If you're an average American, you are probably consuming about 100 g protein (that's way too high) and 5.4 g arginine per day. If you're a heavy meat eater, chances are you're getting quite a bit more arginine to build muscle and to help protect your heart, but also a correspondingly high amount of saturated fat and cholesterol, which endangers your heart. That is why we recommend lean meats, fish, and low-fat cheese as healthy sources in Food Factor 2, the Staminators.

If, on the other hand, you're vegetarian, especially one who eats no eggs or dairy products, you may well be getting inadequate quantities of arginine. At least eight of the amino acids are inarguably essential, which is why pure vegetarians need to take such special pains to make sure a meatless diet doesn't cause a nutritional deficit. Others at risk for arginine deficiency include anyone on a fad diet that allows less than 1,000 calories total per day, and those who stick to a high-carbohydrate, low-fat, and low-protein regimen.

To determine approximately how much arginine you're currently getting from the foods you eat, take a look at the two accompanying charts.

TABLE 5.1

Foods Highest in Arginine

Milligrams per 100 Grams	Food
4,148	Seaweed, spirulina, dried
1,533	Chives, freeze-dried
1,203	Onions, dehydrated flakes
1,042	Soybeans, green, raw

Milligrams per 100 Grams	Food
994	Soybeans, green, cooked, boiled, drained, without salt
994	Soybeans, green, cooked, boiled, drained, with salt
905	Soybeans, mature seeds, sprouted, raw
905	Soybeans, mature seeds, sprouted, cooked, stir-fried
890	Shallots, freeze-dried
859	Peppers, sweet, green, freeze-dried
859	Peppers, sweet, red, freeze-dried
790	Leeks (bulb and lower leaf portion), freeze-dried
658	Spinach, frozen, chopped or leaf, unprepared
648	Mushrooms, shiitake, dried
634	Garlic, raw
629	Cowpeas (blackeyes), immature seeds, frozen, unprepared
629	Soybeans, mature seeds, sprouted, cooked, stir-fried, with salt
627	Peas, mature seeds, sprouted, cooked, boiled, drained, without salt
627	Peas, mature seeds, sprouted, cooked, boiled, drained, with salt
611	Lentils, sprouted, raw
600	Lentils, sprouted, cooked, stir-fried, without salt
600	Lentils, sprouted, cooked, stir-fried, with salt
595	Cowpeas (blackeyes), immature seeds, frozen, cooked, boiled, drained, without salt
595	Cowpeas (blackeyes), immature seeds, frozen, cooked, boiled, drained, with salt
585	Soybeans, mature seeds, sprouted, cooked, steamed, without salt
585	Soybeans, mature seeds, sprouted, cooked, steamed, with salt
561	Spinach, frozen, chopped or leaf, cooked, boiled, drained, without salt
561	Spinach, frozen, chopped or leaf, cooked, boiled, drained, with salt
554	Pepper, ancho, dried
509	Potatoes, mashed, dehydrated, granules with milk, dry form
508	Lima beans, immature seeds, frozen, baby, unprepared

Milligrams per 100 Grams	Food
508	Peppers, hot chili, sun-dried
484	Peas, mature seeds, sprouted, raw
463	Broadbeans, immature seeds, raw
458	Lima beans, immature seeds, raw
456	Lima beans, immature seeds, cooked, boiled, drained, without salt
456	Radishes, Oriental, dried
456	Lima beans, immature seeds, cooked, boiled, drained, with salt
445	Lima beans, immature seeds, frozen, baby, cooked, boiled, drained, without salt
445	Lima beans, immature seeds, frozen, baby, cooked, boiled, drained, with salt
428	Lima beans, immature seeds, frozen, Fordhook, unprepared
428	Peas, green, raw
427	Seaweed, spirulina, raw
423	Peas, green, cooked, boiled, drained, without salt
423	Peas, green, cooked, boiled, drained, with salt
412	Peas, green, frozen, unprepared
407	Peas, green, frozen, cooked, boiled, drained, without salt
407	Peas, green, frozen, cooked, boiled, drained, with salt

www.nutritiondata.com

TABLE 5.2

Average Per Capita Intake of Protein and Arginine in the United States

Source	Estimated Intake	
	Protein	Arginine
	g/d	mg/d
Meat	30.3	2051
Poultry and fish	12.1	680
Dairy products	22.4	720

Source	Estimated Intake	
	Protein	Arginine
	g/d	mg/d
Eggs	6.3	405
Cereals	18.4	762
Other*	10.5	799
Total	100.0	5,417

*The supply of arginine by other foods was calculated by assuming that the percentage contribution to this category was as follows: legumes, 35; nuts and seeds, 35; potatoes and sweet potatoes, 20; fruits, 5; and green and yellow vegetables, 5.

From Visek, 1986. With permission from the American Society for Nutritional Sciences.

If your daily intake of arginine seems on the low side, or if you already suffer from cardiovascular problems, such as hypertension, that increase your body's need for arginine, it may be time to up your daily intake.

IS ARGININE "ESSENTIAL"?

Nutritionists have long classified nutrients as either essential or nonessential. This distinction is misleading, because both categories are equally necessary for good health. Essential nutrients are ones that your body can't produce naturally so it's *essential* that you obtain them from foods or supplements. For example, the body can't synthesize many vitamins. They must be ingested.

Nonessential nutrients, on the other hand, can be produced by your body, and for this reason the Nutrition Council suggests no RDA—or recommended daily allowance—for them. Getting these nutrients from your diet is nonessential because your body can make what it needs—*assuming you aren't consuming too few calories for healthy functioning.*

Arginine falls into a gray area: Some nutritionists classify it as essential, while others argue that it is nonessential. It is true that the body can make arginine. The controversy lies in whether or not we can make enough of it to meet our needs. A highly respected medical textbook, *Pathological Physiology,* 6th edition, by Drs. Sodeman and Sodeman (1979), concluded that we often can't make it ourselves—and thus classified arginine as essential.

A WORD OF CAUTION ABOUT ARGININE

Herpes simplex virus (HSV) is currently the most common sexually transmitted disease in the United States. For this reason, we feel it is necessary to point out that in some people diagnosed with herpes, a high-arginine diet may provoke a flare-up or outbreak of blisters. HSV responds well to increased lysine. To see a complete reference table of lysine to arginine ratios, visit http://www.herpes.com/nutrition.shtml.

Also, people with certain kinds of cancer or at high risk for cancer may wish to consult their physician about the advisability of a high-arginine diet: Depending on the type of tumor, high-arginine diets have been shown to both reduce tumors and promote their growth (Yeatman, Risley, and Brunson, 1991; Bronte, Kasic, et al., 2005).

COMMON FACTOR 2 FOODS

We've outlined common high-arginine foods and provided some description of their nutritional properties below.

Nuts

The evidence is overwhelming that dietary nut consumption promotes sexual vitality directly by supplying arginine-derived nitric oxide—1 cup of almonds, for instance, supplies more than 3,535 mg arginine. A comparable portion of top sirloin beefsteak provides less than half that amount of arginine.

Nuts and seeds also promote sexual vitality indirectly because they are antioxidants that can significantly lower the LDL cholesterol that was shown in a previous section to jeopardize sexual vitality (Jenkins, Kendall, et al., 2003).

Nuts have also been shown to help promote weight loss when eaten in moderation (Alper and Matte, 2002), help reduce the risk for diabetes (Jiang, Manson, et al., 2002), and reduce the risk of heart disease.

In the early 1990s, more than thirty-one thousand Seventh Day Adventists in Loma Linda, California, participated in a study of diet and coronary heart disease (CHD) risk. Subjects who ate nuts one to four times each week had a 27 percent reduced risk of dying from heart disease compared with those who ate nuts less than once per week. Those who ate nuts five or more times each week cut their risk of death from heart disease by nearly half (48 percent) even after adjusting for the conventional risk factors—age, smoking, exercise, and high blood pressure. It was observed that those who ate nuts daily lived on the average nearly three years longer than those who seldom ate nuts (Fraser, Sabate, et al., 1992).

Researchers from the Harvard School of Public Health likewise concluded that regular consumption of nuts reduces the risk of coronary heart disease (Hu, Stampfer, et al., 1998). Nuts are good for you for the following reasons:

- Nuts are high in fat, but the fat is mostly healthy unsaturated fat.

- Almonds especially, but also walnuts, significantly lower blood cholesterol levels.

- Nuts have a high arginine content, needed to produce NO.

- Nuts are high in alpha-linolenic acid, an essential (n-3 or omega-3) fatty acid.

- Nuts are also good sources of dietary fiber, magnesium, copper, folic acid, vegetable protein, potassium, and vitamin E.

Although nuts are high in fat, the Adventist health study reported that those participants who frequently ate nuts were actually leaner than those who didn't eat nuts. Similar observations were made in other reports on nut consumption (Fraser, 1999).

The Physicians' Health Study, as reported in *Archives of Internal Medicine*, also showed in more than twenty thousand participants that regularly consuming nuts significantly lowered the risk of heart disease and death (Albert, Gaziano, et al., 2002). Those who consumed a serving of nuts (about 1 ounce) twice a week or more were 47 percent less likely to suffer sudden cardiac death than those who seldom or never ate nuts.

Nuts, especially almonds, are featured in the Harvard *Healthy Eating Pyramid* (Willett, 2001). Almonds have also been shown to be as effective in lowering cholesterol as drug therapy with lovastatin (Jenkins, Kendall, et al., 2003). For readers being treated for high cholesterol, this is not a suggestion to discontinue your prescribed medication; we do, however, encourage you to discuss adding nuts to your diet with your medical health care practitioner.

Here is a nutritional breakdown of commonly available nuts:

• **Almonds,** 1 cup whole kernels, dry-roasted, no salt added: 30 g protein, 3,535 mg arginine, 824 calories, 73 g total fat, zero cholesterol, 1 mg sodium.

• **Brazil nuts,** 1 cup, dried, unblanched, shelled: 20 g protein, 3,007 mg arginine, 918 calories, 93 g total fat, zero cholesterol, 4 mg sodium.

• **Cashews,** 1 cup, dry-roasted, no salt added, halves and wholes: 21 g protein, 2,385 mg arginine, 786 calories, 63 g total fat, zero cholesterol, 22 mg sodium.

• **Chestnuts** (European variety), 1 cup, roasted: 5 g protein, 325 mg arginine, 350 calories, 3 g total fat, zero cholesterol, 3 mg sodium.

• **Coconut,** 1 cup, raw, shredded: 3 g protein, 437 mg arginine, 283 calories, 27 g total fat, zero cholesterol, 16 mg sodium.

• **Filberts (hazelnuts),** 1 cup, raw, chopped: 17 g protein, 2,543 mg arginine, 722 calories, 70 g total fat, zero cholesterol and sodium.

• **Macadamia nuts,** 1 cup, raw, halves or whole: 11 g protein, 1,879 mg arginine, 962 calories, 102 g total fat, zero cholesterol, 7 mg sodium.

• **Peanuts,*** all types, 1 cup, dry-roasted, no added salt: 35 g protein, 4,134 mg arginine, 854 calories, 73 g total fat, zero cholesterol, 9 mg sodium.

• **Peanut butter,** 2 tablespoons, chunky-style, no salt added: 8 g protein, 920 mg arginine, 188 calories, 16 g total fat, zero cholesterol, 5 mg sodium.

• **Pecans,** 1 cup, raw, chopped: 10 g protein, 1,283 mg arginine, 753 calories, 78 g total fat, zero cholesterol and sodium.

*Peanuts are actually legumes and not nuts, but we include them here. Note that peanuts and foods with some peanut content are a major health concern in the United States, and one of the most common causes of food allergies—especially in children. They account for most of the near-fatal and fatal anaphylactic reactions to foods (Lee and Sheffer, 2003). We advise caution.

- **Pine nuts,** 1 cup, dried: 18 g protein, 3,258 mg arginine, 909 calories, 92 g total fat, zero cholesterol, 3 mg sodium.

- **Pistachios,** 1 cup, raw: 25 g protein, 2,495 mg arginine, 685 calories, 55 g total fat, zero cholesterol, 1 mg sodium.

- **Walnuts** (common English style), 1 cup, chopped: 18 g protein, 2,666 mg arginine, 765 calories, 76 g total fat, zero cholesterol, 2 mg sodium.

Sunflower Seeds

Sunflower seeds are rich in vitamin E as well as in arginine. They are also a good source of folate and other B vitamins and minerals including copper, magnesium, zinc, and selenium. These seeds have become widely popular both as a snack and as an ingredient in baked goods, and even in salads.

- *1-cup serving, hulled, dry-roasted, no salt added: 25 g protein, 2,610 mg arginine, 745 calories, 64 g total fat, zero cholesterol, 4 mg sodium.*

Eggs

Eggs, a staple of breakfast menus, have been on an image roller coaster for years. When Americans began to be cholesterol-conscious, eggs were one of the first foods they stopped eating. In the ensuing years, research has shown that saturated fat has a greater effect on blood cholesterol levels than does dietary cholesterol—and eggs are not a major source of saturated fat.

Eggs acquired a bad reputation when, in the 1970s, the American Heart Association (AHA) suggested restricting their consumption as a way to help limit dietary cholesterol intake to less than 300 mg per day. The AHA has now backtracked; its new guidelines find intake of one yolk a day acceptable, providing other cholesterol-contributing foods are limited in the diet. This restriction is reasonable for people with a history of elevated plasma cholesterol or established coronary heart disease, but may be overly restrictive for people without these conditions. In healthy individuals, the nutritional benefits of an egg may actually outweigh the concern about the cholesterol it holds.

In a recent study that examined the food intake of 117,000 nurses and health professionals over a fourteen-year period, no difference was found in the relative risk for CHD between those who consumed less than one egg per week and those who ate more than an egg a day, with the exception of those with diabetes (Hu, Stampfer, et al., 1999).

The *Journal of the American College of Nutrition* reported that in "free living" populations, as compared with "laboratory populations," egg consumption is not associated with higher cholesterol levels (Kritchevsky, 2004). An earlier report in the same journal stated, "When dietary confounders were considered, no association was seen between egg consumption at levels up to 1+ egg per day and the risk of coronary heart disease in non-diabetic men and women" (Kritchevsky and Kritchevsky, 2000).

As a whole food, eggs supply all sorts of goodies, including folate, riboflavin, selenium, choline, and vitamins B_{12}, A, K, and D. Egg whites are a source of high-quality protein, and the lipid complex in the yolk enhances the bioavailability of antioxidant nutrients such as lutein and zeaxanthin (see chapter 6).

Lecithin is an essential component of all biological membranes, modulating the activation of membrane enzymes such as superoxide dismutase (SOD). Choline, a component of egg lecithin, is essential for normal development of the brain. It has numerous important physiological functions. Eggs are one of the few foods that contain high concentrations of choline (Zeisel, Mar, et al., 2003).

The color of the shell, or for that matter the color of the yolk, has no bearing on egg quality or nutritional value. Duck, goose, or quail eggs are available at some gourmet shops or local farms.

A word of caution: In recent years, poisoning caused by salmonella bacteria has raised health concerns about eggs. In the past, this occurred only when salmonella bacteria in chicken intestines penetrated the egg through a crack in the shell. More recently, however, salmonella bacteria have been found in clean uncracked eggs. Therefore, washing eggs before cracking them and observing other careful handling techniques may not be enough to protect you from infection. To safeguard your health, the eggs must be cooked at sufficiently high temperatures to destroy the bacteria. Undercooked egg dishes, such as soft-cooked or sunny-side-up fried eggs, or recipes made with raw eggs like Caesar salad dressing and eggnog, carry the risk of salmonella infection.

Since there is still some controversy over the contribution of eggs' cholesterol to either health or disease, it might be wise to consider what dietary measures can be implemented as a safeguard should this confer even a small risk. A high-ORAC antioxidant intake immediately comes to mind (see chapter 6).

- *1-cup serving, whole, cooked, hard-boiled, or chopped: 17 g protein, 1,027 mg arginine, 211 calories, 14 g total fat, 577 mg cholesterol, 169 mg sodium.*

- *1-cup serving, whole, cooked, scrambled: 24 g protein, 1,417 mg arginine, 365 calories, 27 g total fat, 774 mg cholesterol, 616 mg sodium. (Scrambled eggs provide about a 40 percent increase in cholesterol and a 70 percent increase in sodium for a 30 percent gain in arginine.)*

Fish

Fish provide an excellent low-fat source of protein, as well as the n-3 (omega-3) polyunsaturated fatty acids (PUFAs) found in fish oil. Consuming fish oil improves endothelial function, leading directly to the enhancement of NO production (Chin and Dart, 1995; Harris, Rambjor, et al., 1997).

N-3 fatty acids are anticoagulant: They reduce the likelihood that blood platelets will cling to blood vessel walls (Abe, El-Masri, et al., 1998). They also affect the production of inflammatory agents such as the interleukins and other molecules believed to play a role in atherosclerotic plaque formation (Carter, 2005).

Omega-3 PUFAs have triglyceride-lowering properties (Grimsgaard, Bonaa, et al., 1997). In a comprehensive review of human studies, it was reported that approximately 4 g per day of omega-3 fatty acids from fish oil decreased serum triglyceride concentrations by 25 to 30 percent, with accompanying increases in LDL cholesterol of 5 to 10 percent, and in HDL cholesterol of 1 to 3 percent (Harris, 1997).

Nonetheless, studies on the dietary benefits of fish are somewhat mixed. Epidemiological studies show that men and women who eat at least some fish weekly have a lower incidence of coronary heart disease than those who don't (Hu, Bronner, et al., 2002; Stone, 1996). On the other hand, the US Physicians' Health Study failed to find such an association (Ascherio, Rimm, et al., 1995).

It is important to look at the details of scientific studies when interpreting the results. In one study, only survivors were evaluated, and it is conceivable that individuals who did not survive ate less fish. Another explanation, based on a rigorous analysis of a number of cohort studies, is that the protective effect of fish consumption depends on the CHD risk status of the population studied, with some people being at greater risk than others. Another consideration relates to the type of fish consumed—fatty versus lean (Marckmann and Gronbaek, 1995).

We recommend eating fish in moderation as a good way to increase intake of omega-3 fatty acids while also increasing arginine. All fish contain the omega-3 acids EPA and DHA—they are our major source for these. However, the concentrations vary from one species to another in accordance with their feed and whether wild-harvested or farm-raised. Farm-raised catfish, for instance, tend to have less EPA and DHA than do wild catfish, whereas farm-raised salmon and trout contain similar amounts to their wild counterparts.

The Food and Nutrition Board, Institute of Medicine, and National Academies, in collaboration with Health Canada, released the Dietary Reference Intakes for Energy and Macronutrients in 2002. The acceptable range for alpha-linolenic acid is estimated to be 1.3 g to 2.7 g per day on the basis of a 2,000-calorie diet. This is ten times the current intake of EPA+DHA.

These recommendations can easily be met by following the AHA Dietary Guidelines to consume two fish meals per week, with an emphasis on fatty species—salmon, herring, and mackerel—and by using liquid vegetable oils containing alpha-linolenic acid. Commercially prepared fried fish from restaurants and fast-food establishments, as well as many frozen, convenience-type fried fish products, should be avoided because they are low in omega-3 and high in trans-fatty acids. The growing popularity of sushi, raw fish on a pillow of rice and seaweed, is helping many people include more fish in their diet.

In the United States, people consume most omega-3 fatty acids in the form of alpha-linolenic acid in EPA and DHA. The major food sources of alpha-linolenic acid are vegetable oils, principally canola and soybean oils.

Other food sources that are rich in alpha-linolenic acid include flaxseed (23 g per 100 g) and English walnuts (7 g per 100 g). See table 5.3.

TABLE 5.3
α-Linolenic Acid Content of Selected Vegetable Oils,
Nuts, and Seeds

Food	α-Linolenic Acid Content, g/tbsp
Olive oil	0.1
Walnuts, English	0.7
Soybean oil	0.9
Canola oil	1.3
Walnut oil	1.4
Flaxseeds	2.2
Flaxseed (linseed) oil	8.5

Adapted from USDA Nutrient Data Laboratory, www.nalusda.gov/fnic/foodcomp/, accessed October 3, 2002.

A Word About Fish Oil Supplements

Fish oil supplementation of more than 3 g EPA+DHA per day should be done only under medical supervision. The Food and Drug Administration (FDA) has noted that a greater daily intake could result in excessive bleeding in some individuals (Office of Nutritional Products, 2002). The cardio-protective benefit of eating fish is achieved with a considerably lower intake of 1 g per day, which has almost no potential for adverse effects.

Fish oil has also been shown to lower blood pressure (Morris, Sacks, et al., 1993), but the American Heart Association does not recommend this as a sole treatment given the high doses required. Other nutritional modifications (such as salt restriction and increased fruit and vegetable consumption) and antihypertensive medications work better.

In 1997, the FDA ruled that dietary intakes of up to 3 g per day of marine omega-3 fatty acids are generally recognized as safe (GRAS).

Safety of Fish

Some species of fish may contain significant levels of mercury, polychlorinated biphenyls (PCBs), dioxins, and other environmental contaminants. These substances are present at low levels in fresh waters and oceans, and they can concentrate in the aquatic food chain such that levels are generally highest in older, larger predatory fish and marine mammals.

Fish and seafood are a major source of human exposure to these contaminants. PCBs and methylmercury have long half-lives in the body and can accumulate in people who consume contaminated fish on a frequent basis. We recommend eating deep-water fish to keep mercury consumption to a minimum.

Consumers can reduce their exposure to PCBs by removing the skin and fat from these fish before cooking them; however, because methylmercury is distributed throughout the muscle, skinning and trimming does not significantly reduce mercury concentrations in fillets.

The Environmental Protection Agency (EPA) advises pregnant women, those who may become pregnant, and nursing mothers to limit their consumption of sport-caught fish to one 6-ounce meal per week. The EPA also recommends that young children consume less than 2 ounces of sport-caught fish per week, and that women who are pregnant or nursing and young children eliminate shark, swordfish, king mackerel, and tilefish (also referred to as golden bass or golden snapper) from their diets completely while limiting their consumption of other fish to 12 ounces (three to four servings) per week to minimize exposure to mercury. The EPA's lists of fish advisories can be found on its website: www.epa.gov/waterscience/fish.

The FDA has concluded that aside from pregnant women and women who may become pregnant, it's safe to consume up to 7 ounces per week of fish with mercury levels around 1 part per million (ppm)—shark, swordfish, king mackerel, tilefish—and 14 ounces a week of fish with mercury levels averaging 0.5 ppm (fresh tuna, orange roughy, marlin, red snapper). Information currently available about the methylmercury content of selected fish can be found on the FDA website: www.cfsan.fda.gov/~frf/sea-mehg.html.

Fatty Fish

So-called fatty fish are highest in the cardioprotective fish oils described above. These fish have a "fishier" taste, as a result of the higher oil concentration.

TABLE 5.4

Fish: A Quick Reference Guide

Lean	Moderate Fat	High Fat
Black sea bass	Barracuda	Herring
Brook trout	Striped bass	Butterfish
Cod	Swordfish	Mackerel
Haddock	Trout	Salmon
Hake	Tuna	Smelt
Halibut	Whiting	Sturgeon
Ocean perch		Yellowtail
Red snapper		
Rockfish		
Tilapia		

Mackerel

An oily fish related to tuna, mackerel, too, has outer layers of red meat and lighter interior meat. All types of mackerel are higher-fat fish and rich in omega-3 fatty acids. Most of the commercial catch is canned, but fresh mackerel is also available from the waters off California as well as the eastern coasts of the United States and South America. Fresh mackerel is very perishable and must be handled with special care. This fish is marketed dressed or in fillets, and can be poached, baked, or broiled.

- *4.5-ounce serving, Atlantic, raw: 21 g protein, 1,247 mg arginine, 230 calories, 16 g total fat, 78 mg cholesterol, 101 mg sodium.*

Salmon

Salmon are rich in omega-3 fatty acids that help fight heart disease by lowering triglyceride levels and making the blood less likely to clot. Omega-3 fatty acids found mainly in fish also seem to lessen symptoms of rheumatoid arthritis and can lower blood pressure. Canned salmon is a good source of B vitamins, and the cooked, edible bones furnish a significant amount of the calcium helpful in preventing osteoporosis.

- *8-ounce serving, Atlantic, farmed, raw: 39 g protein, 2,358 mg arginine, 362 calories, 21 g total fat, 117 mg cholesterol, 117 mg sodium.*

- *6-ounce serving, coho, farmed, raw: 34 g protein, 2,024 mg arginine, 254 calories, 12 g total fat, 81 mg cholesterol, 75 mg sodium.*

- *16.5-ounce serving, sockeye, canned, without salt, drained solids with bone: 76 g protein, 4,520 mg arginine, 565 calories, 27 g total fat, 162 mg cholesterol, 277 mg sodium.*

- *18-ounce serving, pink, canned, without salt, solid with bone and liquid: 90 g protein, 5,375 mg arginine, 631 calories, 27 g total fat, 250 mg cholesterol, 340 mg sodium.*

Tuna

People consume more tuna than any other type of fish in this country. About 95 percent is sold canned. A large saltwater fish, tuna has deep red and dense flesh. It is meaty, soft, and looks almost like beef when raw; it firms up and turns lighter in color when it is cooked. Fresh tuna should be reddish and not brown when it is purchased. It's most commonly sold in steaks or slices; it can be marinated and then grilled, poached, baked, broiled, or sautéed.

- *3-ounce serving, fresh, bluefin, raw: 20 g protein, 1,187 mg arginine, 122 calories, 4 g total fat, 32 mg cholesterol, 33 mg sodium.*

- *7-ounce serving, white, canned in water, without salt, drained solids: 41 g protein, 2,430 mg arginine, 220 calories, 5 g total fat, 72 mg cholesterol, 86 mg sodium.*

Lean Fish

Lean fish are a very healthful alternative to red meat. Low in fat and calories, but rich in high-quality protein, lean fish are a good source of vitamin E (a major antioxidant nutrient) and omega-3 fatty acids. Although fatty fish have more omega-3 fatty acids than lean fish, even lean fish are a good source—and these healthful fatty acids are found in very few other foods.

Lean fish typically have a mild flavor, easily adaptable to a wide range of cuisines. These white-meat fish are sufficiently similar in taste and texture that you can substitute one variety for any other.

Catfish

This tasty freshwater fish, once common only in the South, is now one of America's favorite fish, thanks to fish farming. The fish has a smooth but tough skin that can be difficult to remove, so it is preferable to buy fillets or nuggets.

- *6.5-ounce serving, channel, wild, raw: 26 g protein, 1,558 mg arginine, 151 calories, 4 g total fat, 92 mg cholesterol, 68 mg sodium.*

Cod

Cod is firm, white, and mild, great for chowders and stews. Small cod, less than 3 pounds, are sometimes marketed as scrod, which are sweeter and more tender than full-grown cod.

- *8-ounce serving, Atlantic, raw: 41 g protein, 2,463 mg arginine, 189 calories, 2 g total fat, 99 mg cholesterol, 125 mg sodium.*

Flounder

Mild flavor and light texture make this a popular choice. The winter flounder from New England is sometimes called lemon sole; other flounders are offered as gray sole and petrale sole. Dover sole is either imported from England or a type of Pacific flounder that is sometimes called sole in the United States. Flounder is sold whole, dressed or filleted, fresh and frozen.

- *3-ounce serving (flounder and sole), raw: 10 g protein, 638 mg arginine, 52 calories, zero total fat, 28 mg cholesterol, 46 mg sodium.*

Groupers

Various species known as groupers are marketed under that name. Red and black groupers are taken from South Atlantic waters and the Gulf of Mexico. They may weigh from 3 to 20 pounds when sold fresh as steaks or fillets.

- *9-ounce serving, mixed species, raw: 50 g protein, 3,002 mg arginine, 238 calories, 3 g total fat, 96 mg cholesterol, 137 mg sodium.*

Haddock

A smaller version of the cod, this lean North Atlantic fish can be substituted for cod in most recipes.

- *7-ounce serving, raw: 36 g protein, 2,183 mg arginine, 168 calories, 1 g fat, 110 mg cholesterol, 131 mg sodium.*

Halibut

A flatfish like flounder, halibut can be found in both North Atlantic and North Pacific waters. It's a very large fish, usually marketed in fillets or steaks, more commonly frozen than fresh.

- *7-ounce serving, Atlantic or Pacific, raw: 42 g protein, 2,540 mg arginine, 224 calories, 5 g total fat, 65 mg cholesterol, 110 mg sodium.*

Mahimahi

This is the Hawaiian name for a fish that is also called dolphin or dolphin-fish, although it's unrelated to dolphins (porpoises). Caught primarily in Pacific waters, it is most often sold in fillets or steaks, fresh or frozen, with the skin attached to hold the fish together during cooking. Despite its rich, sweet flavor, mahimahi is a lean fish.

- *7-ounce serving, raw: 38 g protein, 2,258 g arginine, 173 calories, 1 g total fat, 149 mg cholesterol, 180 mg sodium.*

Pollack

Mild white Alaska pollack from the Pacific are commonly made into fish sticks and surimi (mock crabmeat). Atlantic pollack is a different species, richer and more flavorful. Though sometimes called Boston bluefish, it is not related to true bluefish. It has a dark layer of flesh just under the skin on one side, which can be removed for a milder flavor.

- *7.6-ounce serving, Atlantic, raw: 38 g protein, 2,246 mg arginine, 178 calories, 2 g total fat, 137 mg cholesterol, 166 mg sodium.*

Sea Bass

This is a category of lean saltwater fish, suitable for almost any method of cooking. Giant sea bass are members of the grouper family. Chile is the main supplier of this family of fish.

- *4.5-ounce serving, mixed species, raw: 24 g protein, 1,423 mg arginine, 125 calories, 3 g total fat, 53 mg cholesterol, 88 mg sodium.*

Snapper

Red snapper, caught off the southeastern coast of the United States, is by far the best-known snapper and is in great demand. Its bright red skin is usually left on the fillets to identify it.

- *8.6-ounce serving, mixed species, raw: 45 g protein, 2,675 mg arginine, 218 calories, 3 g total fat, 81 mg cholesterol, 139 mg sodium.*

Swordfish

A large saltwater fish with meaty, rich-tasting flesh, swordfish can be found off both US coasts. Swordfish is usually sold in boneless loins (a lengthwise quarter section of the whole fish), steaks, or chunks, fresh or frozen.

- *5.4-ounce serving, raw: 27 g protein, 1,612 mg arginine, 165 calories, 5 g total fat, 53 mg cholesterol, 122 mg sodium.*

Trout, Freshwater

Trout are related to salmon; whole trout may range from 1½ to 10 pounds. Rainbow trout, the most commonly available, is sold fresh or frozen throughout the country all year. Only farm-raised rainbows are sold commercially.

- *2.8-ounce serving, farmed, raw: 16 g protein, 987 mg arginine, 109 calories, 4 g total fat, 47 mg cholesterol, 28 mg sodium.*

Shellfish

Shrimp

Shrimp ranks second to tuna as Americans' favorite seafood. Like chicken, the dense white meat of shrimp has a fresh, mild flavor that goes well with many ingredients. You can buy shelled and cleaned (deveined) shrimp or even precooked shrimp to use as a quick, convenient (and considerably more expensive) recipe ingredient. Almost all shrimp caught are frozen at sea for optimal freshness, then thawed for sale, or sold frozen (thawed shrimp should be labeled "previously frozen"). Shrimp are low in fat and calories, but higher in cholesterol than most seafood.

- *28 g (4 large), raw: 6 g protein, 497 mg arginine, 30 calories, zero total fat, 43 mg cholesterol, 41 mg sodium.*

Lobster

The king of crustaceans, lobsters contain sweet, firm, succulent meat within their claws, tail, and body cavity. They must be cooked alive or killed just before they are cooked.

- *150-g serving (1 lobster), northern, raw: 28 g protein, 2,463 mg arginine, 135 calories, 1 g total fat, 142 mg cholesterol, 222 mg sodium.*

- *8-g serving spiny lobsters, mixed species, raw: 43 g protein, 3,760 mg arginine, 234 calories, 3 g total fat, 146 mg cholesterol, 370 mg sodium.*

Crayfish

These crustaceans are found in freshwater lakes, streams, and rivers in Louisiana and some other parts of the country, particularly the Pacific Northwest. They are also farmed in several Southern states. Harvested at about 5 inches long, they're most commonly cooked live and served whole like lobster or crab. The meat tastes somewhat like lobster, although less dense and rich. Crayfish are sold live or fresh frozen, and the tails are also sold cooked. Unlike most other shellfish, crayfish (and shrimp) have a relatively high cholesterol content, with about 178 mg in a 3.5-ounce serving of cooked crayfish.

- *3-ounce serving, mixed species, farmed, raw: 13 g protein, 1,101 mg arginine, 61 calories, 1 g total fat, 91 mg cholesterol, 53 mg sodium.*

Meat

As mentioned earlier, meat is a rich source of arginine, but it can also contribute a large amount of fat and cholesterol to the diet. We balance out our plan with the high antioxidant values found in Factor 3 Foods (the Brights), but we suggest selecting meats that are as lean as possible, whenever possible. Fresh meat is better for people with high blood pressure because it does not have the high sodium content of processed meat (luncheon meat, hot dogs, sausages, canned ham, and the like).

Beef

The per capita beef consumption in the United States is steadily declining due to concerns about levels of saturated fat and cholesterol, its role in obesity and heart disease, and, to some extent, fear of mad cow disease. Due to consumer preference for low-fat protein, ranchers are crossbreeding traditional breeds with leaner, larger cattle, feeding cattle more grass and less corn, and sending younger livestock to market. Meatpackers and retailers are trimming more external fat, leaving about 0.1 inch, down from .75 inch just five years ago.

Beef can be a part of a low-fat diet if you follow three simple steps: Choose lean cuts, eat small portions (3.5 to 4 ounces, cooked), and trim all visible fat before cooking. With these precautions, beef is an excellent source of iron, zinc, and vitamin B_{12}—nutrients that can be difficult to obtain elsewhere, certainly not from a vegetarian diet. You don't need to eat slabs of steak or roast to get the nutritional benefits beef has to offer, and trimming the fat has no effect on meat's nutrient value.

Fat content in beef varies widely depending on the cut. Consider two factors when choosing a low-fat cut of beef: grade and cut. Grading is a voluntary service established by the USDA and offered to slaughterhouses: Government inspectors evaluate beef carcasses for marbling, the white streaks or specks of fat within the flesh itself that help give meat its juiciness and distinct flavor. Ironically, the system rewards the production of fatty beef: The cuts with the most marbling are given the highest grade, *Prime,* followed by *Choice* and *Select.* In 1987, to make lean beef more appealing to consumers, the USDA coined the term *Select* to replace the category *Good.*

On average, a cut of beef graded Select has 5 to 20 percent less fat than Choice beef of the same cut, and 40 percent less fat than Prime beef. Since grading is not compulsory and is an added expense to the meatpacker, much of the beef in the supermarkets is ungraded—about 44 percent in 1989, according to the American Meat Institute. This ungraded beef is usually of Choice or Select quality and may be sold under the store's brand name. Choice is the most common designation of the beef that is graded.

Cut, the part of the animal from which a piece of meat is taken, is perhaps more important than grade when determining fat content. Select beef of one cut may have more fat than Choice beef of another. For example, 3.5 ounces of Select trimmed blade roast (chuck) has 14 g fat, compared with 6 g fat in 3.5 ounces of Choice trimmed top round.

• **Brisket,** 3-ounce serving, whole, separable, lean only, all grades, raw: 18 g protein, 1,110 mg arginine, 168 calories, 6 g total fat, 54 mg cholesterol, 66 mg sodium.

• **Bottom sirloin,** 4-ounce serving, tri-tip roast, separable lean and fat, trimmed to zero fat, all grades, raw: 21 g protein, 1,335 mg arginine, 164 calories, 9 g fat, 65 mg cholesterol, 52 mg sodium.

• **Chuck, blade roast,** 3-ounce serving, separable lean and fat, trimmed to 0.1 inch fat, prime, raw: 24 g protein, 876 mg arginine, 278 calories, 24 g total fat, 63 mg cholesterol, 54 mg sodium.

• **Chuck, ground,** 3-ounce serving, 80 percent lean meat and 20 percent fat, pan-broiled patty (hamburger): 20 g protein, 1,347 mg arginine, 231 calories, 14 g total fat, 73 mg cholesterol, 71 mg sodium.

• **Eye round,** 3-ounce serving, separable lean and fat, trimmed to 0.13 inch fat, all grades, raw: 18 g protein, 1,179 mg arginine, 141 calories, 6 g total fat, 36 mg cholesterol, 48 mg sodium.

• **Flank,** 4-ounce serving, separable lean and fat, trimmed to zero fat, all grades, raw: 21 g protein, 1,372 mg arginine, 155 calories, 7 g total fat, 35 mg cholesterol, 54 mg sodium.

• **Rib eye,** 3-ounce serving, small end (ribs 10 to 12), separable lean and fat, trimmed to zero fat, Choice (Delmonico), raw: 15 g protein, 942 mg arginine, 233 calories, 19 g total fat, 58 mg cholesterol, 48 mg sodium.

• **Shank, crosscuts,** 3-ounce serving, separable lean and fat, trimmed to 0.25 inch fat, Choice, raw: 18 g protein, 1,101 mg arginine, 150 calories, 9 g total fat, 36 mg cholesterol, 51 mg sodium.

• **Short loin, top loin,** 3-ounce serving, separable lean only, trimmed to 0.13 inch fat, Choice, raw: 18 g protein, 1,248 mg arginine, 132 calories, 6 g total fat, 57 mg cholesterol, 48 mg sodium.

• **Tenderloin,** 3-ounce serving, separable lean and fat, trimmed to 0.25 inch fat, Prime, filet mignon, beef medallion, raw: 15 g protein, 660 mg arginine, 240 calories, 21 g total fat, 60 mg cholesterol, 42 mg sodium.

- **Top round,** 3-ounce serving, separable lean and fat, trimmed to 0.13 inch fat, all grades, London broil, minute steak, round steak, raw: 18 g protein, 1,209 mg arginine, 141 calories, 29 g fat, 257 mg cholesterol, 51 mg sodium.

- **Veal,** 3-ounce serving, breast, whole, boneless, separable lean and fat, raw: 15 g protein, 873 mg arginine, 177 calories, 12 g total fat, 60 mg cholesterol, 60 mg sodium.

Our list would not be complete without the "All-American" hot dog, without which there would never have been such a thing as a baseball game:

- **Frankfurter,** 2-ounce hot dog (aka frank and wiener), cooked: 6 g protein, 404 mg arginine, 169 calories, 15 g total fat, 29 mg cholesterol, 600 mg sodium.

Lamb

Today's lamb is lean, thanks to extensive trimming of its external fat; on average, only 0.25 inch or less is left on retail lamb. Like beef, lamb is graded for quality. The same category names are used—*Prime* and *Choice*—but these terms do not indicate the same differences in fat content as they do in beef. The majority of lamb to reach the market is Choice, which, nutritionally, is comparable to Choice beef: Many corresponding cuts contain the same amount of internal fat and offer similarly significant levels of protein, zinc, riboflavin, and vitamin B_{12}.

- **Foreshank,** 3-ounce serving, separable lean and fat, trimmed to 0.13 inch fat, Choice, raw: 15 g protein, 954 mg arginine, 171 calories, 12 g total fat, 60 mg cholesterol, 60 mg sodium.

- **Ground,** 3-ounce serving, raw: 15 g protein, 825 mg arginine, 240 calories, 21 g total fat, 63 mg cholesterol, 51 mg sodium.

- **Leg and shoulder cubed for stew or kebab,** 3-ounce serving, separable lean only, trimmed to 0.25 inch fat, raw: 18 g protein, 1,017 mg arginine, 114 calories, 3 g total fat, 54 mg cholesterol, 54 mg sodium.

- **Leg, shank half,** 3-ounce serving, separable lean and fat, trimmed to 0.13 inch fat, Choice, raw: 15 g protein, 636 mg arginine, 171 calories, 12 g total fat, 57 mg cholesterol, 48 mg sodium.

- **Rib,** 3-ounce serving, separable lean and fat, trimmed to 0.13 inch fat, Choice, raw: 12 g protein, 858 mg arginine, 282 calories, 30 g total fat, 63 mg cholesterol, 48 mg sodium.

Pork

Pork has suffered for years from a reputation as a high-fat meat, in large part because many pork products such as sausage do include a good deal of fat. Yet recent research has shown that, in many cases, "fat as a pig" is no longer an accurate statement. Improved ways of breeding, feeding, and raising pigs mean that fresh pork, on average, is now 31 percent lower in fat, 29 percent lower in saturated fat, 14 percent lower in calories, and 10 percent lower in cholesterol than it was several decades ago. This has led to its new identity as "the other white meat."

Pork is not as lean as skinless turkey or chicken breast or lean fish, and only the leanest cuts approach the low fat content of these meats. Other lower-fat cuts are comparable to the leanest cuts of beef. Still, pork is an excellent source of B vitamins and is the leading food source of thiamin, a B vitamin necessary for the conversion of carbohydrates into energy and important for normal functioning of the cardiovascular and nervous systems. Pork also supplies good amounts of iron, zinc, and high-quality protein. Moreover, the fat in pork is slightly less saturated than that in beef.

Unlike the case of beef, there is no reliable grading system for pork to give a clue to the fat content of the cut. Still, because fresh pork is consistent in quality, no grading system is needed.

- **Leg (ham),** 3-ounce serving, whole, separable lean and fat, raw: 15 g protein, 948 mg arginine, 207 calories, 15 g total fat, 63 mg cholesterol, 39 mg sodium.
- **Sirloin,** 1 chop, boneless, separable lean and fat, raw: 21 g protein, 1,336 mg arginine, 151 calories, 7 g total fat, 67 mg cholesterol, 52 mg sodium.

Poultry

Many consumers now make a conscious decision to eat less red meat and more poultry in an effort to lower dietary fats. When cooked, light-meat chicken without the skin is 33 to 80 percent leaner than trimmed cooked beef, depending on the cut and grade of the beef. Chicken breast, the leanest part of the chicken, has less than half the fat of a trimmed Choice-grade T-bone steak and chicken fat is less saturated than the fat found in beef.

Chicken and Cornish Hens

• **Chicken, broilers or fryers, light meat, meat only,** raw, 100-g serving (3.5 ounces): 23 g protein, 1,399 mg arginine, 114 calories, 2 g total fat, 58 mg cholesterol, 68 mg sodium.

• **Chicken, broilers or fryers, light meat, meat and skin,** raw, 100-g serving (3.5 ounces): 20 g protein, 1,268 mg arginine, 186 calories, 11 g total fat, 67 mg cholesterol, 65 mg sodium.

• **Chicken, broilers or fryers, dark meat, meat only,** raw, 100-g serving (3.5 ounces): 20 g protein, 1,211 mg arginine, 125 calories, 4 g total fat, 80 mg cholesterol, 85 mg sodium.

• **Chicken, broilers or fryers, dark meat, meat and skin,** raw, 100-g serving (3.5 ounces): 17 mg protein, 1,053 mg arginine, 237 calories, 18 g total fat, 81 mg cholesterol, 73 mg sodium.

• **Cornish game hen, meat only,** raw, 100-g serving (3.5 ounces): 17 g protein, 1,078 mg arginine, 200 calories, 14 g total fat, 101 mg cholesterol, 61 mg sodium.

Duck

• **Duck, domesticated, meat and skin,** raw, 100-g serving (3.5 ounces): 11 g protein, 770 mg arginine, 404 calories, 39 g total fat, 76 g cholesterol, 63 mg sodium.

Goose

• **Goose, domesticated, meat and skin,** raw, 100-g serving (3.5 ounces): 16 g protein, 987 mg arginine, 371 calories, 34 g total fat, 80 mg cholesterol, 73 mg sodium.

Turkey

Tradition regards turkey as a once-a-year, Thanksgiving treat. Most—about 90 percent—are sold during November and December. They are large birds and sometimes too much to handle as a staple food. But today, health-conscious people are making turkey a part of their regular diet. As a result, turkeys are now produced in greater numbers and are available in many forms, in contrast with a few years ago, when they were mostly available whole.

Consumers can select the parts they prefer, such as whole or half breasts, cutlets, and tenderloins; these cook much faster than a whole bird.

Turkey breast is the leanest of all meats, supplying less than half a gram of fat per 3-ounce serving, skinned. Even *with* skin, a 3-ounce serving derives only 18 percent of its calories from fat. The dark meat is higher in fat than the light meat, yet still relatively lean if eaten without the skin, deriving only about 34 percent of its calories from fat. It is an excellent source of protein, B vitamins (niacin and B_6), phosphorus, selenium, and zinc. It also has some iron, riboflavin, and magnesium.

• **Turkey, fryer-roaster, breast, meat and skin,** raw, per 100-g serving (3.5 ounces): 24 g protein, 1,669 mg arginine, 125 calories, 3 g total fat, 70 mg cholesterol, 48 mg sodium.

• **Turkey, young hen, breast, meat and skin,** raw, per 100-g serving (3.5 ounces): 20 g protein, 1,421 mg arginine, 168 calories, 9 g total fat, 63 mg cholesterol, 61 mg sodium.

• **Turkey, fryer-roaster, leg, meat only,** raw, per 100-g serving (3.5 ounces): 20 g protein, 1,420 mg arginine, 108 calories, 2 g total fat, 84 mg cholesterol, 71 mg sodium.

• **Turkey, fryer-roaster, leg, meat and skin,** raw, per 100-g serving (3.5 ounces): 20 g protein, 1,412 mg arginine, 118 calories, 4 g total fat, 87 mg cholesterol, 69 mg sodium.

• **Turkey, young hen, leg, meat and skin,** raw, per 100-g serving (3.5 ounces): 19 g protein, 1,364 mg arginine, 151 calories, 8 g total fat, 63 mg cholesterol, 70 mg sodium.

• **Turkey, ground,** raw, per 100-g serving (3.5 ounces): 17 g protein, 1,204 mg arginine, 149 calories, 8 g total fat, 79 mg cholesterol, 94 mg sodium.

Game

Certain game birds are becoming popular, due to the relatively low cholesterol values per portion.

• **Ostrich, ground,** raw, per 100-g serving (3.5 ounces): 20 g protein, 1,383 mg arginine, 165 calories, 9 g total fat, 72 mg cholesterol, 72 mg sodium.

6

Factor 3 Foods—The Brights

Stop, Thief! You Stole My Electron!

Oxygen molecules (O_2) are typically made up of two atoms held together in a particular pattern or configuration by a force called a chemical bond consisting of pairs of electrons. When a bond breaks, the molecule is fragmented and each part is left with an unpaired electron. These molecular fragments are the notorious free radicals. They have a high electrical charge and are chemically unstable.

"Unstable" here means that they will bounce around with great energy and break up other bonds, "stealing" their electrons and, thus, giving up their own chemical freedom. We call this process oxidation. Chemical misery loves company: When free radicals break bonds, the process can cascade into a chain reaction of broken bonds and more liberated free radicals.

FREE RADICAL ASSASSINS

Science coined the term *oxidative stress* to describe the damage that free radicals resulting from body activity do to our organs, cells, and tissues. Little stands in the way of free radicals in the mad scramble of oxidation.

They'll damage cell membranes and blast chunks out of DNA. No cells or other parts of the human body are exempt from free radical attack, but five key body structures are particularly vulnerable to free radical oxidative damage: cell membranes, mitochondria, DNA, enzymes, and fat (www.renewalsresearch.com). Here's what free radicals can do to the body:

- Interfere with cell membrane function and impair their metabolism and waste removal.
- Damage mitochondria, the cell powerhouses, and thus impair metabolic energy production.
- Damage DNA, which can interfere with normal cell reproduction and is now thought to be a leading cause of cancer.
- Oxidize low-density lipoprotein (LDL) cholesterol, the body's "bad cholesterol," which can cause atherosclerosis (hardening of the arteries).

Free radicals are a normal by-product of metabolism, but there are many factors that will increase their production beyond ordinary levels, including:

- Poor diet.
- Stress.
- Prolonged strenuous exercise.
- Food additives.
- Alcohol.
- Herbicides.
- Hydrogenated vegetable oils.
- Air and water pollutants.
- Foods that are barbecued, fried, grilled, or otherwise cooked at high temperatures.
- Radiation.

Metabolic stress is caused by free radical buildup from both ordinary and extraordinary activities of our body. When we are more active, the free radical buildup increases accordingly. With each increase in activity, our body needs to eliminate free radicals as soon as possible because they attack everything in sight. Our cardiovascular system, blood vessels, and heart are some of the targets for free radicals.

There are others. For instance, exposure of naked skin to the ultraviolet radiation in sunlight causes free radical formation in the skin. This breaks down collagen support and causes wrinkling and accelerated skin aging. Also, the free radicals that form when your eyes are exposed to bright light increase the incidence of "age-related" macular degeneration. This is why health-care practitioners urge us to avoid sunbathing and to wear tinted lenses when outdoors.

As noted earlier, free radicals readily attach to LDL cholesterol (LDL-C), causing the cholesterol to become oxidized. Oxidized LDL-C is taken up by immune system macrophage (Greek for "large eaters") cells and transported into our blood vessel walls, where it begins to form atherosclerotic plaque.

Free radicals can cause blood platelets to stick together in the bloodstream, thus "thickening" it. Free radicals can also cause all sorts of cells in the bloodstream to stick to the walls of the blood vessels, impeding blood flow.

Free radicals damage DNA at the cellular level, attacking the structures called mitochondria—cellular power plants. The job of the mitochondria is to convert organic material into energy in the form of ATP. Free radical damage to the mitochondria has recently been linked to accelerated aging (Dizdaroglu, Jaruga, et al., 2002).

The average body cell DNA is bombarded with about ten thousand free radical "hits" per day. With advancing age, the hit rate rises to about two million per day. Since metabolism continuously generates free radicals, we want to eliminate as many hits as possible, as quickly as possible. Luckily, many of our body organs and cells—especially in the cardiovascular system—*can* rejuvenate after free radical damage, and keeping that damage to a minimum helps reduce aging.

Significantly reducing daily food intake is one way to reduce metabolic free radical formation, but for most of us this is not a realistic strategy. Also, as we mentioned above, food is not the only source of free radicals: Lengthy unprotected exposure to sunlight increases free radical formation and has been strongly linked to melanoma skin cancer (Haywood, Wardman, et al., 2003). Fortunately, we have a more enjoyable alternative: In-

creased consumption of dietary antioxidants (especially carotenoids—
see page 117), primarily in the form of delicious fruits and vegetables, can
protect us against that risk (Sies and Stahl, 2004).

Free radical cell DNA damage can be assessed in the body by measuring the excretion of a by-product of DNA repair (8-oxo-7,8-dihydro-2'-
deoxyguanosine). We know the rate at which the body excretes this by-
product when it is under free radical attack, so we can measure the change
in that rate of excretion after eating particular foods.

It turns out that brussels sprouts actually are exceptionally good for
you—300 g (about 1⅓ cups) of brussels sprouts daily will reduce the excretion rate by about 28 percent (Verhagen, Poulsen, et al., 1995).

It is important to eat antioxidant foods on a daily basis, not just for
sexual health but for the health of the entire body. DNA damage occurs
on a daily basis, and when not repaired, various tissues can become
damaged—in particular, the endothelium. This can lead to cardiovascular and heart disease, sexual dysfunction, accelerated aging, and, in some
people, cancer.

Scientists think that free radical tissue damage is the underlying mechanism of many diseases; epidemiological studies have shown that in countries where the diet is rich in antioxidant foods, the rate of these diseases is
significantly lower. The "Mediterranean diet" eaten in Greece and Italy
is antioxidant-rich.

It is estimated that only 10 percent of the US population consumes five
servings of fruits and vegetables per day, as recommended by the American
Cancer Society.

THE SEXUAL COST OF FREE RADICALS

Free radicals can be found throughout the body searching for a chemical
home such as LDL-C globules. They can infiltrate various cell membranes
until they find a host to which they can attach, damaging it in the process.
As free radicals combine with LDL-C, the vascular system sustains damage, impairing the ability of the endothelium to provide the nitric oxide
(NO) critical to sexual function. Antioxidants offer powerful protection
against this impairment (Catapano, 1997).

Research has shown that an eight-week regimen of antioxidants—in this case derived from the polyphenols in a certain species of brown algae—significantly improved erectile function (Kang, Park, et al., 2003). The Brights are common foods, primarily fruits and vegetables, that contain powerful antioxidants (far tastier than brown algae).

ANTIOXIDANT SUPERHEROES

The body needs to protect itself with free-radical-scavenging antioxidants. Antioxidants are substances that prevent or slow the process of oxidation. Known as free radical scavengers, antioxidants are substances that neutralize O_2 free radicals and prevent them from attacking your body.

Approximately 4 percent of the O_2 you breathe converts to free radicals in your body, mostly as a result of ordinary metabolism. Concentration of more than 21 percent free radicals in your body can result in serious tissue injury. That's what happens in an atomic radiation "burn."

Even the "good" oxygen that we breathe in deeply during aerobics classes is actually a toxic gas, even though our body depends on it for life. Remember, when iron is exposed to oxygen, it rusts.

A tragic example of the toxicity of oxygen was the discovery that when premature infants were given pure oxygen in incubators to help them breathe, the treatment blinded many of them. Fortunately, nature has provided us with a built-in mechanism that regulates the amount of oxygen our body can tolerate to the volume needed for ongoing activity, plus a very small reserve—merely a few minutes' worth. Nature needed to compromise, gambling that most of us will be able to get fresh oxygen within a few minutes, avoiding the risk of "rusting."

It is oxidation that causes an apple pulp to turn brown shortly after it has been bitten into. But if lemon juice is applied to it, it will retain its whitish color. In this case, ascorbic acid in the lemon juice is antioxidant. Potatoes also become brown when they are skinned. Commercial antioxidants prevent browning, giving potato chips that well-known and appealing pale yellow color.

Our red blood cells (erythrocytes) contain a molecule called hemoglobin that transports oxygen. Hemoglobin is red by virtue of the iron it contains, and it's programmed to limit oxygen concentration in the blood by a finely tuned physiological mechanism involving cooperation between the lungs and the kidneys. If that mechanism failed us and the gas volume of oxygen in our body rose above a certain level, our tissue would actually burn up. Too much oxygen is as hazardous as too little of it.

The human body produces its own antioxidant—in particular the enzyme superoxide dismutase (SOD). Even the amino acid arginine, a component of protein, is an antioxidant, but the body depends heavily on external dietary sources for antioxidant substances. These include vitamins C and E from fresh fruits and vegetables, the polyphenols and proanthocyanidins in red and yellow fruits and vegetables, the tannins in wine, tomatoes, and grape seed extract (oil) and olive oil. These are major potential antioxidant dietary sources. Antioxidants are listed in *Great Food, Great Sex* by food type.

ORAC: THE RUST PREVENTION INDEX

In 1993, researchers from the Jean Meyer USDA Human Nutrition Research Center on Aging at Tufts University in Boston reported the development of an oxygen-radical absorbance capacity (ORAC) technique that permits determining how many free radicals a given amount of an antioxidant food can actually absorb (Cao, Alessio, and Cutler, 1993). It would be music to the ears of the senior President Bush to learn that half a cup of blueberries—even frozen berries—beats a cup of broccoli by a country mile.

The procedure used to determine an ORAC value is rather complex. It involves an elaborate chemical comparison of the laboratory preparation of a given food sample with a chemically irradiated analog of vitamin E called trolox. Trolox has a known O_2 free radical absorption rate, and trolox absorption units can be converted to ORAC units.

One ORAC unit has the capacity to neutralize approximately one hundred million O_2 free radicals per second.

Table 6.1 gives ORAC-unit values for specified quantities of given foods. We have also converted the ORAC units to approximate vitamin C equivalents so that you can determine about how much vitamin C you would have to consume to meet that ORAC antioxidant value.

TABLE 6.1

ORAC Value of Dietary Antioxidants in Common Foods

Food	ORAC units/100 g	ORAC serving size	ORAC/ serving	Vitamin C equivalent mg/serving
BERRIES				
Raisins	2,830	¼ cup	1,019	1,925.9
Blueberries	2,400	½ cup	1,620	3,061.8
Blackberries	2,036	½ cup	1,466	2,770.7
Strawberries	1,540	½ cup	755	1,427.0
Raspberries	1,227	½ cup	755	1,427.0
Cranberries	1,150	½ cup	831	1,571.0
FRUITS				
Prunes	5,770	1 prune	462	873.2
Cantaloupe	2,520	½ melon	670	1,266.3
Plums	949	1 plum	626	1,183.1
Orange	750	1 orange	182	344.0
Grapes (red)	739	10 grapes	177	334.5
Cherries	670	10 cherries	455	860.0
Kiwi	605	1 fruit	458	865.6
Grapefruit	483	½ fruit	580	1,096.2
Grapes (white)	446	10 grapes	107	202.2
Banana	221	1 banana	300	567.0
Apple	218	1 med. apple	300	567.0
Apricot	164	3 raw	175	330.8
Peach	158	1 med.	137	259.0
Pear	134	1 med.	222	419.6
Watermelon	100	1 cup (154 g)	154	291
Honeydew melon	97	1 cup (177 g)	172	325
CHOCOLATE				
Chocolate (dark)	13,120	1 piece (50 g)	6,560	12,398
Chocolate (milk)	6,740	1 piece (50 g)	3,370	637
VEGETABLES & LEGUMES				
Red beans	11,459	1 cup (177 g)	20,282	20,282.4
Wheat bran	4,620	1 cup (47.2 g)	2,171	4,104.0

Food	ORAC units/100 g	ORAC serving size	ORAC/ serving	Vitamin C equivalent mg/serving
Garlic	2,000	1 clove	58	109.6
Kale	1,770	½ cup, cooked	1,150	2,173.5
Spinach	1,260	1 cup	678	1,281.4
Cabbage (red)	1,000	1 cup (150 g)	1,500	2,835
Brussels sprouts	980	1 sprout	206	389.3
Alfalfa sprouts	930	1 cup	307	580.2
Broccoli florets	890	½ cup, cooked	817	1,544.1
Beets	850	½ cup, cooked	715	1,351.4
Avocado	782	½ Florida avocado	49	281.6
Pepper (red bell)	731	1 med. pepper	540	1,020.6
Onion	450	½ cup, chopped	360	680.4
Corn	400	½ cup, cooked	330	623.7
Peas (frozen)	400	½ cup	291	550.0
Eggplant	390	½ cup, cooked	185	349.7
Cauliflower	377	½ cup, cooked	188	355.3
Sweet potato	300	½ cup, cooked	301	568.9
Potato	300	½ cup, cooked	244	416.2
Cabbage	300	½ cup, raw	105	198.5
Leaf lettuce	262	10 leaves	200	378.0
Kidney beans	250	½ cup, cooked	400	756.0
Lettuce	250	10 leaves	200	378.0
Tofu	213	½ cup	195	368.6
Carrot	207	½ cup, cooked	160	302.4
Tomato	200	1 med. tomato	233	440.4
Green (string) bean	200	½ cup	125	236.3
Carrot	200	½ cup, raw	115	217.4
Zucchini	176	½ cup, raw	115	217.4
Squash (yellow)	150	½ cup, cooked	183	345.9
Lima beans	136	1 cup (178 g)	77	144.4
Lettuce (iceberg)	100	5 large leaves	116	219.2
Celery	100	½ cup, diced	60	113.4
Cucumber	100	½ cup, slices	28	52.9

Adapted from: http://optimalhealth.cia.corn.com.au/OracLevels.htm

	ORAC per 100 g	Serving size	ORAC per serving
NUTS & SEEDS			
Walnuts	6,153	1 cup (117 g)	5,259
Sunflower seeds	1,582	1 cup, hulled (128 g)	1,236
Hazelnuts	147	1 cup (115 g)	128
Almonds	88	1 cup (145 g)	61

	Serving size	ORAC per serving
Red wine (generic)	1 glass (3.5 fl oz, fl 103 g)	679.6

	ORAC per 100 g	Serving size	ORAC per serving
Wheat bran	4,620	1 cup (47.2 g)	2,180.6

STANDARD ANTIOXIDANTS	
Ascorbate	442,000
Trolox	400,000
Vitamin E	201,000

Adapted from Medallion Laboratories, Analytical Progress, Summer 2001, Vol. 19, No. 2. (9000 Plymouth Ave North, Minneapolis, Mn 55427; (763) 764–4453; see info@medlabs.com)

TABLE 6.2

ORAC value of polyphenols, flavonoids, and catechins

The ORAC-units value of wines and tea may be given in some instances, but it is more common to simply state that their high antioxidant action is due to their high contents of polyphenols, catechins and bioflavonoids (these terms are explained elsewehere). Rarely is the consumer informed about how, exactly, antioxidant they are:

Catechin	ORAC per 100 g
Gallic acid	15,900
Epigallocatechin	15,000
Epicatechin	23,100
Epicatechin gallate	23,500
Gallocatechin gallate	14,000
Epigallocatechin gallate	17,900
Quercetin	22,200
Kaempherol	9,100
Naringenin	8,800
Ascorbic acid	6,800

Adapted from Henning, Fajardo-Lira, et al., 2003. Reprinted with permission from Lawrence Erlbaum Associates.

Researchers from the US Department of Agriculture (USDA) center who developed the ORAC scale have recommended about 5,000 ORAC units per day to maintain health. It is estimated that the average American daily ORAC-unit intake is about 1,750. You would have to take 3,061.8 mg of vitamin C to get the antioxidant equivalent of the 1,620 ORAC units in half a cup of blueberries.

PUT MORE POWER ON YOUR PLATE

There has been an explosion of antioxidant supplements in the health food market. Why not just take a handful of pills to protect your DNA? In addition to missing out on the fun and flavor of wholesome foods, supplements may not be the best way to get your daily antioxidant dose. If you think you can easily meet your antioxidant needs by consuming vitamin supplements, think again.

The ORAC equivalent of the recommended daily dosage of a popular brand of vitamin supplement sold nationwide is 88.5. To meet the 5,000-ORAC-unit daily criterion for maintaining health, you would have to consume 56.5 times the recommended daily dosage . . . each day.

The *Los Angeles Times* (October 27, 2003) summarized the effect of antioxidant supplementation on a sample of more than twenty thousand British adults cited in a study by Canoy, Wareham, et al. The article reported that ". . . people who took antioxidant supplements received no greater protection from chronic diseases than those who didn't." This prompted Melanie Polk, M.S., R.D., director of nutrition education at the American Institute of Cancer Research, to add, "We should be spending our money in the produce department, not the vitamin aisle."

We definitely agree. Great food, like great sex, is the way to go.

Nutritional scientists are increasingly comfortable in recommending a diet rich in fruits and vegetables to help reduce the risk of hypertension, cardiovascular disease (CVD), and cancer. We recommend the same diet to restore, protect, and enhance sexual performance.

The Brights are rich in the most powerful antioxidants that nature provides, and studies have shown that supplementing with vitamins such as E and C does not result in a significant decrease in the excretion of the DNA repair by-product. Whatever it is in fresh fruits and vegetables that is antioxidant, it must be something other than the conventional vitamins E, C, and beta-carotene (Cao, Russell, et al., 1998). In fact, it has been found that more than 80 percent of the total antioxidant capacity of fruits and vegetables comes from constituents other than vitamins (Wang, Cao, and Prior, 1996).

The great news is that we have recently discovered the crucial role antioxidants play in protecting—even enhancing—the health and function of the sex organs as well as the associated reproductive organs crucial for sexual vitality. This is why the Brights have such an integral role in the healthy eating plan of *Great Food, Great Sex*.

FOLLOW THE RAINBOW

Nutrient chemicals in plants are called phytochemicals. The nutrients in the Brights belong to a group called polyphenols, and a staggering number of different types exist—perhaps more than eight thousand. They are the most abundant group of plant (phenol) compounds, and they account for the flavor, color, and taste of fruits, vegetables, seeds, and their other consumable parts. This is why they are referred to as "rainbow foods."

Antioxidant polyphenols have been shown to help decelerate the aging process, help protect the major organs in the body, and in general contribute to improved health. Antioxidant nutrients help us stay young and healthy. Without this heroic protection against the relentless attack of free radicals, we would rust on the inside, develop disease, and die younger.

Polyphenols are the major elements of the plant world immune system. In order for plants to thrive, they must protect themselves from insects, bacteria, and molds. They do this by producing substances that are either distasteful and/or toxic to predators.

In concentration, these substances often don't taste too good to people, either, and they are usually bitter. Many foods contain tannins, plant polyphenol substances somewhat bitter to the taste. They were once called "antifeedants" because they seem in a sense to be the plant's effort at avoiding being consumed. In condensed form, these tannins are called proanthocyanidins.

These polyphenols have antioxidant, anti-inflammatory, antiallergenic, and, in many instances, antibacterial properties. In a recent study, ten different plant polyphenols were evaluated and found to inhibit some varieties of foodborne bacteria such as *Staphylococcus aureus, Salmonella, Escheria coli,* and others. The antioxidants included epigallocatechin and black and green tea polyphenols (Taguri, Tanaka, and Kouno, 2004).

By helping protect us against free radicals, the polyphenols serve as preventive medicine for cardiovascular diseases, cancer, and many other ailments—and, of course, for sexual dysfunction.

Plant polyphenols also confer indirect benefits on sexual vitality: The enzyme 5-alpha-reductase inhibits the conversion of testosterone to its more potent form, 5-alpha-dihydrotestosterone. That form of testosterone is responsible for the benign prostatic enlargement (BPH) that begins to plague men in their midfifties, interfering with proper urinary flow. It is also thought to be a possible precursor of hormone-dependent prostate cancer in many men.

In its benign form, BPH may also jeopardize sexual vitality because a number of prescription medications used to treat BPH interfere with sexual function, and surgery for BPH has the potential to damage nerves, leading to impotence. It has been shown in clinical studies that polyphenols in saw palmetto naturally inhibit 5-alpha-dihydrotestosterone, and saw palmetto continues to be studied as an alternative treatment for BPH (Hiipakka, Zhang, et al., 2002).

Consider tomatoes, a star member of the Brights. Research has shown that tomato products are a source of lycopene, shown to reduce the risk of prostate cancer (Campbell, Canene-Adams, et al., 2004). In many cases, nutrients can be destroyed by cooking, but lycopene is best liberated by cooking tomatoes. Spaghetti sauce is a great source of lycopene.

Multidrug prostate and breast cancer treatment is often thwarted by a particular protein in the body that prevents transport of the drugs to the cancer. Polyphenols have been shown to reduce that resistance to the drug treatments (Cooray, Janvilisri, et al., 2004). Black tea polyphenols were also shown to be beneficial in prevention of hormone-dependent human breast tumors (Way, Lee, et al., 2004).

MYSTERIOUS ANTIOXIDANTS CURED "THE SCORBUT"

In the winter of 1534–1535, Jacques Cartier was exploring the St. Lawrence River region of Canada with an expeditionary force of more than one hundred men. The winter was harsh, and the men were seriously ill. His diary described the symptoms of scurvy—then known as scorbut—as the principal cause of the men's severe illness, and they were facing death.

Cartier consulted natives of the region, who directed him to boil the red bark lining from a particular pine tree and have his men drink this concoction. They recovered within a week. They had consumed powerful super antioxidants that we now call OPCs (oligomeric proanthocyanidins), one of a class of bioflavonoids now sold here and in Europe in health food stores and pharmacies in the United States as pycnogenol (Schwitters and Masquelier, 1993).

Upon his return to France, Cartier promptly reported his finding to the royal court, and his annals were duly remitted to the royal library and . . . forgotten. But more than two hundred years later, the British naval surgeon James Lind (1716–1794) proposed that sailors consume oranges, rich in bioflavonoids, to stave off scurvy. However, oranges were too sour for their tastes, so they boiled them in sugar—reducing the bioflavonoid concentration, but in the process inventing marmalade.

A recent study demonstrated that pycnogenol may actually do considerably more than stave off scurvy. As we explained earlier, an erection requires the relaxation of the arterial smooth muscles in the penis in order to allow increased blood inflow. The trigger for this event is the production of nitric oxide (NO) by the endothelium in the blood vessels as well as by the endothelium lining the spongy cavernosal erectile chambers in the penis. Ordinarily, NO is synthesized from the amino acid arginine. Pycnogenol is known to significantly increase NO production.

Forty men ages twenty-five through forty-five years old, with erectile dysfunction of unknown origin, received the equivalent of 1.7 g (1,700 mg) arginine in a drinkable solution for a period of three months. During the second month, they received a supplementary 40 mg pycnogenol twice per day. During the third month, the dosage of pycnogenol was increased to 40 mg three times per day.

After one month of treatment with arginine only, the results were negligible (5 percent restoration of erectile function). But after the second month with the combination of arginine and pycnogenol, restoration of erectile function rose to 80 percent. After the third month of treatment, 92.5 percent of the men experienced normal erection. No adverse side effects were noted (Stanislavov and Nikolova, 2003).

Pycnogenols also help to prevent age-related diseases such as atherosclerosis due to their antioxidant protection of the vascular endothelium (Fitzpatrick, Bing, and Rohdewald, 1998; Liu, Lau, et al., 2000).

ANTIOXIDANTS 101

As suggested by their name, the Brights are easily recognized by their vibrant color, ranging from deep green to bright red, orange, and yellow. The Brights can add almost endless flavor and variety to every meal, as well as make any dish more visually appealing.

Lycopene is the red carotenoid found in tomatoes, red grapefruit, apricots, and watermelon. This antioxidant has been the subject of much recent research showing its value in cancer prevention.

Indole carbinol 3 and sulforaphane stimulate the production of cancer-killing enzymes. They are plentiful in brussels sprouts, kale, collard greens, broccoli, mustard greens, cabbage, and cauliflower.

Vitamin C, found in citrus fruits, tomatoes, potatoes, peppers, and broccoli, has been said to be the primary water-soluble antioxidant in the body. We cannot produce vitamin C internally and so must obtain it from food and supplemental sources.

Carotenoids are a form of vitamin A derived from plant products. They are pigments synthesized by the action of the sun (photosynthesis). There are more than six hundred carotenoid antioxidants, the major one of which is beta-carotene. Vitamin A is derived from beta-carotene in the liver. It stimulates production of white blood cells and helps maintain skin, respiratory tract surfaces, mucous membranes, and secretions. Sources of beta-carotene include carrots, cantaloupe, and most other yellow, orange, and red fruits and vegetables.

Dark green vegetables such as broccoli, romaine lettuce, and spinach are also good sources—the darker color indicates a higher beta-carotene content. All the carotenoids, including those that cannot be converted to vitamin A, can also bind to oxygen radicals and serve as antioxidants under certain conditions.

Lutein and zeaxanthin help prevent degeneration of the macula, the surface inside the eye that contains the cells needed for vision. Dark green leafy vegetables are the primary source of lutein and zeaxanthin, but colorful fruits and vegetables, such as broccoli, orange peppers, corn, peas, persimmons, and tangerines, also contain these antioxidants.

Beta-1,3-D-glucan, a polysaccharide (sugar) found in maitake mushrooms, stimulates the immune system's natural killer cells and macrophages.

The anti-aging antioxidant ellagic acid is found in grapes, wine, berries, walnuts, apples, tea, and pomegranates.

Flavonoids (also known as bioflavonoids) comprise the most abundant group of plant polyphenols next to phenolic acids. They include resveratrol, found in red wine, and the lignans in nuts, seeds, and grains. Flavonoids, as antioxidants go, are especially kind to the endothelium.

Resveratrol suppresses the growth of Ishikawa (endometrial cancer) cells by inhibiting tumor growth (Kaneuchi, Sasaki, et al., 2003), while epigallocatechin, plentiful in green tea, inhibits the growth of cervical tumor cells (Sah, Balasubramanian, et al., 2004).

Green vegetables, especially leafy ones, contain the polyphenols known as proanthocyanidins, among the most powerful antioxidants that nature produces. When their green color changes to one of the rainbow colors, these compounds become anthocyanidins.

If an apple a day keeps the doctor away, it is most likely due to quercetin, a flavonoid building block for other flavonoids that are abundant in black and green tea. Like other antioxidants, it fights cardiovascular and heart diseases. But it also enhances NO production by the endothelium when taken in combination with grape seed extract, a good source of anthocyanidins, thus supporting sexual vitality (Clifton, 2004).

COMMON FACTOR 3 FOODS: VEGETABLES

Here is a selection of vegetables in the Brights.

Beets

Beets have the highest sugar content of any vegetable, but they are very low in calories. Their sweet flavor comes through even if the beets are canned; most beets are sold that way. Fresh beets, however, have twice the folic acid and potassium, and are crisp in texture.

- *1-cup serving, raw: 2 g protein, 57.1 mg arginine, 58 calories, zero total fat, 106 mg sodium.*

Bell Peppers, Green

These bell-shaped vegetables are sweet bell peppers in their mature green stage when they are fully developed, but not ripe. As they ripen on the vine, most bell peppers turn red and become sweeter. Green bell peppers are excellent sources of many essential nutrients, especially vitamin C.

- *1-cup serving, chopped, raw: 1 g protein, 64 mg arginine, 30 calories, zero total fat, 4 mg sodium.*

Bell Peppers, Red

Red bell peppers are sweet, juicy, colorful, nutritious, and excellent sources of many essential nutrients. By weight, red peppers have three times as much vitamin C as citrus fruit. Moreover, red peppers are a good source of beta-carotene, fiber, and vitamin B_6.

- *1-cup serving, chopped, raw: 1 g protein, 71.5 mg arginine, 39 calories, zero total fat, 3 mg sodium.*

Cabbage, Red

Red cabbage, a member of the large family of cruciferous vegetables, is rich in nutrients, indoles, dietary fiber, and vitamin C (supplying almost twice as much vitamin C as green cabbage).

- *1-cup serving, raw, shredded: 1 g protein, 66.7 mg arginine, 19 calories, 0.2 g total fat, 8 mg sodium.*

Carrots

Carotenoids, the group of plant pigments of which beta-carotene is a member, are so named because they were first identified in carrots. This ever-popular vegetable is also a source of disease-fighting flavonoids, and carrots contain a specific type of fiber, called calcium pectate, that may lower blood cholesterol. With the exception of beets, carrots contain more sugar than any other vegetable, which makes raw carrots a satisfying snack. Some of the nutrients in carrots are more easily absorbed when the vegetable has been cooked even briefly.

- *1-cup serving, raw, shredded: 1 g protein, 61.4 mg arginine, 47 calories, 0.2 g total fat, 39 mg sodium.*

Corn

Corn is a high-carbohydrate food that is metabolized as a starch, so it is not the best choice if you are trying to lose weight. In the United States, each year we eat about 25 pounds of corn per person. Recent developments in corn genetics have produced varieties called supersweet that have more than twice the sugar content of regular corn.

- *1-cup serving, raw: 16 g protein, 780 mg arginine, 606 calories, 8 g total fat, 58 mg sodium.*

Eggplants

For a long time, Americans valued eggplant more as an ornament or table decoration than as a food. It is not high in any single vitamin or mineral. It is very filling, however, while supplying few calories and virtually no fat, and its "meaty" texture makes eggplant a perfect vegetarian main-dish choice. In Italy and France, eggplant is known as aubergine.

- *1-cup serving, raw: 1 g protein, 46.7 mg arginine, 20 calories, zero total fat, 2 mg sodium.*

Leeks

Like onions, to which they are related, leeks are most frequently used to add flavor to various dishes, particularly stews and soups (the best known is vichyssoise, the classic cold potato-and-leek soup from France). Leeks have a milder and sweeter flavor than onions and a crunchy texture when cooked, making them a delicious side dish served on their own. Leeks are surprisingly nutritious, supplying more vitamins and minerals than an equal-sized serving of onions or scallions.

- *1-cup serving, raw: 1 g protein, 69.4 mg arginine, 54 calories, zero total fat, 18 mg sodium.*

Okra

A staple in Southern cuisine, this small green pod is best known as a key ingredient in the thick spicy soup called gumbo. The name is derived from the word *gombo,* which in West African dialect means "okra." The flavor and texture of okra lie somewhere between those of eggplant and asparagus. Cooked okra can be used as a thickener, but some people find the slimy texture unappealing. Sliced and dredged in a light coating of corn-meal, pan-fried okra is crispy with a mild nutty flavor. This unusual vegetable is a good source of vitamin C, folate, and other B vitamins, as well as magnesium, potassium, and manganese. Okra is high in dietary fiber, supplying 4 g per 1 cup cooked.

- *1-cup serving, raw: 2 g protein, 84 mg arginine, 31 calories, zero total fat, 8 mg sodium.*

Onions

Onions are low in calories and in most vitamins and minerals, although they do supply a little calcium, iron, and potassium. However, the many flavorful members of this plant family—including scallions, leeks, shallots, and garlic as well as onions themselves—are rich sources of a number of sulfur compounds that may lower blood pressure and discourage tumor growth; quercetin (a flavonoid with high antioxidant activity); and saponins, which can significantly lower cholesterol.

- *1-cup serving, chopped, raw: 1 g protein, 250 mg arginine, 67 calories, zero total fat and cholesterol, 5 mg sodium.*

Radishes

Radishes are root vegetables and come in many varieties. The most familiar is the red globe radish that pairs juicy crispness with a delicate spicy flavor. The strongest-flavored variety is horseradish, which is grated as a condiment. Radishes also belong to the cruciferous family and were first cultivated thousands of years ago in China, then in Egypt and ancient Greece, where the vegetable was so highly regarded that gold replicas were made of it. As with many other root vegetables, their green tops are edible and lend a peppery taste to salads. Radishes are a good source of vitamin C and make a perfect, very-low-calorie snack food.

- *1-cup serving, sliced, raw: 1 g protein, 46.4 mg arginine, 19 calories, zero total fat, 45 mg sodium.*

Squashes

Squashes are gourds consisting of fleshy vegetable matter protected by a rind. Squashes also include melons and cucumbers. Although some grow on vines and others on bushes, all are commonly divided into one of two main groups, summer and winter. Summer squashes are young plants with soft shells and tender, light-colored flesh. Winter squashes have hard shells and darker, tougher flesh and seeds; they are starchier than summer squashes.

Summer Squashes

These vegetables include zucchini, chayote (rhymes with *coyote*), yellow squash, and pattypan or scallop squash. Most varieties are more than 95 percent water and so offer only a moderate amount of nutrients. The high water content, however, means summer squashes are very low in calories. They can be eaten raw or cooked.

- *1-cup serving, raw: 1 g protein, 56.5 mg arginine, 18 calories, zero total fat, 2 mg sodium.*

Winter Squashes

The more common varieties include Hubbard, acorn squash, butternut, and pumpkin. These may be boiled, baked, or steamed.

- *1-cup serving, raw: 1 g protein, 61.6 mg arginine, 56 calories, zero total fat, 4 mg sodium.*

Sweet Potatoes

Unfortunately, many people eat sweet potatoes only on Thanksgiving. They are among the most nutritious of vegetables. Their bright color is a key to their high beta-carotene content, and they also contain the carotenoids lutein and zeaxanthin. Eaten with the skin, a baked sweet potato is an excellent source of fiber (about half of it is soluble), and they supply substantial amounts of vitamins C and B$_6$, and manganese, as well as a small amount of potassium.

- *1-cup serving, raw: 2 g protein, 102 mg arginine, 114 calories, zero total fat, 4 mg sodium.*

Tomatoes

Fresh tomatoes are a delicious source of vitamin C, and cooked tomatoes contain lycopene, a carotenoid that fights heart disease. Americans eat a lot of tomatoes in processed form such as sauce on pasta or pizza, in soups, stews, and chilies, and as tomato juice. The tomato is more healthful when cooked than when it is raw: Tomatoes contain a lot of water, so they become more concentrated as the water evaporates during cooking. Half a cup of cooked tomatoes in the form of sauce or paste, for instance, is a far more concentrated source of lycopene than half a cup of fresh tomatoes.

Your body absorbs more lycopene from cooked or processed tomatoes, especially when the tomatoes are cooked with a little oil, as they so often are. Serving raw tomatoes with olive oil also enhances lycopene absorption.

- **Tomatoes,** red, ripe, raw, year-round average, per 1 cup cherry tomatoes serving (149 g, 5.3 oz): 18.9 mg vitamin C, 2 g protein, approx. 30 mg arginine, 38 calories, 0.6 g total fat, zero cholesterol, 16 mg sodium.

- **Tomatoes,** orange, raw, per 1 cup, chopped, serving (158 g, 6.2 oz): 25.3 mg vitamin C, 2 g protein, 45.8 mg arginine, zero total fat and cholesterol, 66 mg sodium.

- **Tomatoes, sun-dried, packed in oil,** drained, per 1 cup serving (110 g, 4.3 oz): 112 mg vitamin C, 6 g protein, 135 mg arginine, 234 calories, 15 g total fat, zero cholesterol, 293 mg sodium.

- **Tomatoes, sun-dried,** per 1 cup (54 g, 2 oz): 21.2 mg vitamin C, 8 g protein, 185 mg arginine, 139 calories, 2 g total fat, zero cholesterol, 1131 mg sodium.

- **Tomatoes, crushed, canned,** per 100-g serving (4 oz): 9.2 mg vitamin C, 2 g protein, 38 mg arginine, 32 calories, zero total fat and cholesterol, 132 mg sodium.

- **Tomatoes, canned, pureed,** no salt added, per 1 cup serving (250 mg, approx. 10 oz): 26.5 mg vitamin C, 4 g protein, 80 mg arginine, 95 calories, 1 g total fat, 5 mg cholesterol, 70 mg sodium.

- **Tomato, juice, canned,** no salt added, per serving (243 g, 9.6 oz): 44.5 mg vitamin C, 2 g protein, 36.4 mg arginine, 41 calories, zero total fat and cholesterol, 24 mg sodium.

- **Tomato, soup, canned, condensed,** reduced sodium, per 1 cup serving (224 g, 9.6 oz): 66.4 mg vitamin C, 2 g protein, no value given for arginine, 85 calories, 2 g total fat, zero cholesterol, 49 mg sodium.

- **Tomato soup, canned, condensed,** commercial variety, per 1 cup serving (251 g, approx. 10 oz): 32.4 mg vitamin C, 4 g protein,

120 mg arginine, 151 calories, 1 g total fat, zero cholesterol, 1383 mg sodium.

COMMON FACTOR 3 FOODS: FRUITS

A table, a chair, a bowl of fruit and a violin; what else does a man need to be happy?

—ALBERT EINSTEIN

You don't have to be a genius to appreciate fruits. Fruits are the ultimate dessert. Sweet, refreshing, and virtually fat-free, whole fruits contain a wealth of nutritional goodies including soluble fiber, minerals, vitamins, and powerful antioxidants.

Fruits can be added to your meal plan in many ways—whole, sliced, puréed, or as a colorful garnish. Fruits make a great between-meal snack, and can help with the midafternoon munchies. If your idea of fruit is limited to your breakfast orange juice and the occasional banana, we encourage you to explore this exciting universe of taste, color, and texture.

In the following list, an asterisk indicates an impressively high ORAC-unit value.

Apples

Apples were well established in Greece by at least 800 B.C., and most likely in Italy as well. Apple trees were introduced to Britain in Roman times and from there to North America by settlers in about 1630. Apples come in a wide variety of types, such as Red and Golden Delicious, McIntosh, and Cortland (good for baking). Apples have from about 27 to 300 mg of polyphenol per 100 g fresh weight, depending on the species. Eating 100 g of fresh Red Delicious apple with the skin on provides a total antioxidant activity equal to 1,500 mg vitamin C.

- *1-cup serving, sliced, raw, with skin: 5.1 mg vitamin C, zero protein, 7.5 mg arginine, 65 calories, zero total fat and cholesterol, 1 mg sodium.*

Apricots*

Apricots have a long and distinguished history, supposedly coming to Greece following the invasion of Central Asia by Alexander the Great. In Italy, Pliny referred to the apricot as "the Armenian plum." Around 1540, apricots could be found in English gardens of the aristocracy, from where they were eventually exported to the colonies, and then Australia, South Africa, and New Zealand. Modern apricots are high in vitamin A and can be enjoyed both fresh and dried. One 35-g apricot has 914 International Units of vitamin A.

- *1-cup serving, halves, raw: 15.5 mg vitamin C, 2 g protein, 69.7 mg arginine, 74 calories, 1 g total fat, zero cholesterol, 2 mg sodium.*

Blackberries*

Blackberries provide about 21 mg vitamin C per 100 g. These berries grow wild in brambles—dense bushes with thorns—and have been cultivated relatively recently. Fresh blackberries bruise easily and have a short shelf life, so they should be enjoyed quickly or frozen for later use.

- *1-cup serving, raw: 30.2 mg vitamin C, 2 g protein, no value known for arginine, 62 calories, 1 g total fat, zero cholesterol, 1 mg sodium.*

Blueberries*

The ORAC for blueberries is amazingly high—a quarter cup provides 800 ORAC units (approximately half the ORAC units of five servings of fruits and vegetables) a day. Blueberries are a great choice for sprinkling on your cereal for breakfast.

- *1-cup serving, raw: 14.1 mg vitamin C, 1 g protein, 53.7 mg arginine, 83 calories, zero total fat and cholesterol, 1 mg sodium.*

Cherries*

It is estimated that cherries were probably first cultivated around twenty-five hundred years ago in southern Turkey or Greece. There are two main types, sweet and sour, and they have about 60 to 90 mg of polyphenols per 100 g fresh weight. Cherries have also been shown to be helpful as an anti-inflammatory for joint pain, arthritis, and gout. (Jacob, Spinozzi, et al., 2003).

- *1-cup serving, sweet, raw, without pits: 10.2 mg vitamin C, 1 g protein, 21.1 mg arginine, 74 calories, zero total fat, cholesterol, and sodium.*

Cranberries*

Most Americans only eat cranberries with their turkey at Thanksgiving, or in the form of highly sweetened juice. Cranberries can be stewed with sweet fruits, such as peaches, in compote for a zesty, tart taste and a burst of color. In addition, a health authority in Germany published the recommendation that cranberries be used to treat cystitis (Naber, Ertel, et al., 2003).

- *1-cup serving, raw: 14.6 mg vitamin C, zero protein, 61.6 mg arginine, 51 calories, zero total fat and cholesterol, 2 mg sodium.*

Dates

Dates grow in hot, dry climates, and desert dwellers have relied on their nutrition for centuries. Dates were cultivated in ancient lands from Mesopotamia to prehistoric Egypt, possibly as early as 6000 B.C., and were introduced into California by the Spaniards in 1765. Dried dates are intensely sweet, and make a wonderful snack with a handful of almonds.

- *1 date, Medjool, pitted: zero vitamin C and protein, 18.7 mg arginine, 66 calories, zero total fat, cholesterol, and sodium.*

Figs

Raw figs are deliciously sweet, but not always easy to find. Dried figs are more available, and are a staple in Middle Eastern markets. Figs are an excellent source of calcium, and also contain the antihypertensive phytochemical coumarin. Caution to sun worshipers: Figs hold compounds known as psoralens, which may increase the risk of sunburn (Watemberg, Urkin, and Witztum, 1991).

- *1 large fig, raw: 1.3 mg vitamin C, zero protein, 10.9 mg arginine, 47 calories, zero total fat and cholesterol, 1 mg sodium.*

Grapefruit*

Grapefruit juice contains citrus flavonoid compounds not found in other citrus juices. Naringin is the most prevalent of these and gives grapefruit juice its characteristic bitter taste. Grapefruits were first grown commercially in the West Indies in the 1800s.

- *1-cup serving, raw, pink, red, white, all geographic areas: 79.1 mg vitamin C, 1 g protein, 161 mg arginine, 74 calories, zero total fat, cholesterol, and sodium.*

Grapes*

In 1584, Sir Walter Raleigh landed on what is now the coast of North Carolina. He reported seeing grapes everywhere: ". . . on the sand and on the green soil, on the hills as on the plains, as well as on the tops of tall cedars . . . in all the world the like abundance is not to be found" (www.ars.usda.gov/is/AR/archives/nov97/musc1197.htm).

He was describing native muscadine grapes (*Vitis rotundifolia*), locally called scuppernong. Then, in 1769, Spanish explorers established missions throughout the coastal region of California and planted grapevines with a European variety now known as Mission (a *Vinis vitifera*). In 1839, William Wolfkill planted the first table-grape vineyards in a region of Southern California called Los Angeles. California grapes are now the world's leading fruit industry, reporting average yields of from 25 to 30 tons per hectare.

Grapes contain resveratrol, which has demonstrated both anti-inflammatory and anticancer properties. Red grapes have more resveratrol than green. Dried grapes, or raisins, have the second highest level of antioxidants among fruits and vegetables, but pack a whopping 435 calories per cup.

- *1-cup serving, seedless, red or green (European varieties such as Thompson seedless), raw: 17.3 mg vitamin C, 1 g protein, 208 mg arginine, 110 calories, zero total fat and cholesterol, 3 mg sodium.*

Kiwi Fruit* (Chinese Gooseberry)

Kiwi seeds were introduced to a New Zealand farmer by British missionaries in 1910 and are now a principal crop of that country. Kiwis have a thin, furry brown skin and a beautiful green flesh when sliced open. They are one of the most nutritionally dense foods, providing a higher concentration of vitamins and minerals per calorie than most other fruits, including vitamin C, folate, and potassium.

- *1 kiwi fruit, fresh, raw: 84 mg vitamin C, 2 g protein, 143 mg arginine, 108 calories, 1 g total fat, zero cholesterol, 5 mg sodium.*

Mango*

Mangoes are delicious tropical fruits that are the key ingredient in chutney and East Indian sweet relish. They are a great source of vitamin A, providing 3,894 International Units per 100 g flesh. The skin on mangoes is very thin and is most easily removed with a carrot scraper. The bright orange flesh adds character to traditional fruit salad. Mango is also a great garnish for broiled fish.

- *½-cup serving: 23 mg vitamin C, 0.1 mg vitamin B$_6$, 0.5 g protein, 15.6 mg arginine, 65 calories, zero total fat and cholesterol, 1.5 mg sodium.*

Melons

Melons come in almost as many shapes and sizes as we do. We mention two of the most popular, cantaloupe and honeydew. When melons were first introduced to France around the fifteenth century, one enterprising "foodie" compiled a collection of fifty different ways to enjoy the fruit, ranging from soup to fritters. Most of us today enjoy melons "au naturel" with perhaps a squeeze of fresh lemon. Half a cantaloupe with a scoop of low-fat cottage cheese makes a great quick meal, packed with vitamins C and A, as well as potassium and fiber.

The pale green flesh of the honeydew makes a beautiful contrast when served with cantaloupe on a fruit platter. Try adding melon to your next party tray to complement the cheeses and sliced meats.

- **Cantaloupe**, 3.35-ounce serving: 36.7 mg vitamin C, zero vitamin B$_6$, 1 g protein, 29 mg arginine, 34 calories, zero total fat and cholesterol, 16 mg sodium.

- **Honeydew**, 3.35-ounce serving: 18 mg vitamin C, 6.67 mg vitamin B$_6$, 1 g protein, 14 mg arginine, 36 calories, zero total fat and cholesterol, 18 mg sodium.

Oranges*

The fruit named for its vibrant color inside and out, one orange will meet about 20 percent of an adult's daily folate needs, and it also supplies more than the US recommended daily intake of vitamin C (60 mg for an adult). Eating the whole fruit, rather than simply the juice, also provides fiber. Blood oranges, popular in Europe, have red flesh due to the presence of anthocyanins.

- *1 large orange, raw with peel: 97.9 mg vitamin C, 2 g protein, 153 mg arginine, 107 calories, 1 g total fat, zero cholesterol, 3 mg sodium.*

Peaches*

Fresh peaches are primarily a summer fruit, and nothing rivals their sweet juiciness. White peaches (which look like yellow peaches on the outside) are sometimes available, and these have a denser flesh, similar to a pear. Although peaches originated in China, the Europeans thought the fruit came from Persia and named it *persica*, which means "Persia."

- *1-cup serving, sliced, raw: 11.2 mg vitamin C, 2 g protein, 30.6 mg arginine, 66 calories, zero total fat, cholesterol, and sodium.*

Pears

There are several varieties of pears, but the most common are Bartlett and Bosc. Red pears are also tasty, though not as easy to find. Pears are delicious raw, but also make a nice dessert poached in a little red wine.

- *1 medium pear, raw: 7 mg vitamin C, 1 g protein, 16.5 mg arginine, 96 calories, zero total fat and cholesterol, 2 mg sodium.*

Persimmons

Persimmons are an excellent source of vitamin C, with from 25 to 52 mg per 100 g. They are also very high in tannins and must not be eaten until very ripe and soft. They can often be found in Chinese fruit markets.

- *1 whole persimmon, native, raw: 27 mg vitamin C, zero protein, 8.5 mg arginine, 32 calories, zero total fat, cholesterol, and sodium.*

Pineapple*

Pineapples contain the enzyme bromelain, which seems to have an anti-inflammatory effect. To see if a fresh pineapple is ready to eat, tug on the center leaf of the spiky green top. It should come out easily. Then you can enjoy the real Hawaiian punch.

- *1-cup serving, diced, raw, traditional varieties: 26.2 mg vitamin C, 1 g protein, no value known for arginine, 70 calories, zero total fat and cholesterol, 2 mg sodium.*

Plums*

Fresh plums come in a wide variety of shapes and sizes but offer the most impressive nutritional value when dried into prunes. Prunes have the highest antioxidant value of common fruits and vegetables. Like figs, they also provide calcium.

- *1-cup serving, sliced, raw: 15.7 mg vitamin C, 1 g protein, 14.8 mg arginine, 76 calories, zero total fat, cholesterol, and sodium.*

Pomegranate*

The pomegranate, known as the "jewel of winter," has been the focus of recent nutraceutical research because of its high antioxidant content. Research suggests that pomegranate juice may contain almost three times the total antioxidant capacity as the same quantity of green tea or red wine. It also provides a substantial amount of potassium, is high in fiber, and contains vitamin C and niacin. The whole seeds can be sprinkled on salads and desserts, and used as a garnish for meat, poultry, or fish.

- *1 pomegranate, raw: 9.4 mg vitamin C, 1 g protein, no value known for arginine, 105 calories, zero total fat and cholesterol, 5 mg sodium.*

Raspberries*

Raspberries are a soft, delicate fruit high in fiber and containing vitamin A, folate, antioxidants, and numerous minerals; the juice contains vitamin C, and the seeds contain vitamin E. They tend to be the most expensive of commercially available berries and can be stretched in a mixed berry dish with strawberries and blueberries.

- *1-cup serving, raw: 32.2 mg vitamin C, 1 g protein, no value known for arginine, 64 calories, 1 g total fat, zero cholesterol, 1 mg sodium.*

Strawberries*

Strawberries are high in pantothenic acid, a B vitamin. Half a dozen strawberries provide almost a third of the adult minimum daily requirement. Five strawberries provide more than 50 percent of the minimum daily requirement of vitamin C. Like tomatoes, strawberries have been associated with reduced risk of prostate cancer, but from some phytochemical (as yet unidentified) other than lycopene.
- *1-cup serving, raw: 89.4 mg vitamin C, 1 g protein, 42.6 mg arginine, 49 calories, zero total fat and cholesterol, 2 mg sodium.*

Tangerines* (Mandarin Oranges)

Tangerines are a small, easy-to-peel citrus fruit, high in vitamin C—they provide 920 International Units per 100 g. Tangerines come in a seedless variety that make a great addition to a brown-bag lunch.
- *1-cup serving, raw: 52 mg vitamin C, 2 g protein, 133 mg arginine, 103 calories, 1 g total fat, zero cholesterol, 4 mg sodium.*

Fruit Juices

Whenever possible, try to eat fruits whole, rather than as juice. There are fewer calories; also, valuable fiber is lost in most commercially prepared fruit juices. An exception is fruit concentrate, available in most health food stores. These are in the form of syrups, made from pure fruit, and can be mixed with water or seltzer for a delicious drink with fewer calories than bottled juice.

- **Apple juice,** 9.8-ounce serving, canned or bottled, unsweetened, without ascorbic acid: 2.2 mg vitamin C, zero protein, no value known for arginine, 117 calories, zero total fat and cholesterol, 7 mg sodium.

- **Cranberry juice,*** 10-ounce serving, unsweetened: 23.5 mg vitamin C, 1 g protein, no value known for arginine, 116 calories, zero total fat and cholesterol, 5 mg sodium.

- **Grapefruit juice,*** 9.8-ounce serving, white, unsweetened: 93.9 mg vitamin C, 1 g protein, no value known for arginine, 94 calories, zero total fat and cholesterol, 2 mg sodium.**

- **Orange juice,*** 9.8-ounce serving, includes from concentrate: 124 mg vitamin C, 2 g protein, 77.2 mg arginine, 110 calories, 1 g total fat, zero cholesterol, 2 mg sodium.

- **Pomegranate juice,*** 8-ounce serving, fresh: no value known for vitamin C or arginine, 1 g protein, 140 calories, zero total fat and cholesterol, 30 mg sodium.

- **Prune juice,*** 10-ounce serving: 10.5 mg vitamin C, 2 g protein, no value known for arginine, 182 calories, zero total fat and cholesterol, 10 mg sodium.

- **Tomato juice,*** 9.6-ounce serving, canned without added salt: 44.5 mg vitamin C, 2 g protein, 36.4 mg arginine, 41 calories, zero total fat and cholesterol, 24 mg sodium.

EXTRA ADDED ATTRACTIONS: TEA, WINE, OLIVES AND OLIVE OIL, GRAPE SEED OIL, AND CHOCOLATE

We have now introduced all three Food Factors—but as with many classification systems, there are a few important omissions. In this case, we'd like to add several more excellent sources of antioxidants, including dark chocolate, red wine, and olive oil. Unlike the other members of the Brights, we suggest moderate consumption, but a little does go a long way.

Tea for Two

Tea, especially green tea containing (polyphenol) flavonoids, has been repeatedly shown to protect and improve health. Green tea has been reported in epidemiological studies to inhibit the development of prostate and breast cancers (Gonzales de Mejia, 2003; Mei, Qian, et al., 2004).

**Grapefruit juice can increase the concentration in the body of many prescription medications, ranging from cholesterol-lowering drugs to Viagra. It is prudent to check with your physician to see if any drugs you are taking may fall in this category (*www.heartinfo.org/ms/news/523552/main.html*).

In a study conducted among Asian American (Chinese, Japanese, and Filipino) women in Los Angeles, a significant inverse relationship was found between consumption of black tea—even more so for green tea—and the incidence of breast cancer (Wu, Tseng, et al., 2003).

Green tea is rich in catechin polyphenols, particularly epigallocatechin gallate (EGCG), a powerful antioxidant. EGCG has been shown to inhibit the growth of cancer cells, and kills cancer cells without harming healthy tissue. It has also been effective in lowering LDL cholesterol levels and inhibiting the abnormal formation of blood clots, or thrombosis, the leading cause of heart attacks and stroke.

A study conducted in 1997 at the University of Kansas showed that EGCG is twice as powerful as resveratrol, the polyphenol found in red wine. This may help explain the relatively low rate of heart disease among Japanese men despite high rates (approximately 75 percent) of smoking.

Green tea is increasingly being promoted as a weight-loss aid, and is definitely a better choice than diet soda. Remember, there is caffeine in green tea, though less than in black tea and coffee. Green tea also kills the bacteria that cause dental plaque. So put the kettle on and pour yourself (and your partner) a nice cup of tea: The mild flavor makes it more palatable unsweetened than black tea, but if you want it sweeter, try stirring in a teaspoon of your favorite honey. You may also enjoy iced green tea, also available by the can or bottle in many Japanese food stores and take-out restaurants.

TABLE 6.3

ORAC Values for Tea

	ORAC Units per 1-Cup Serving
Bigelow Green Tea	1,477
Lipton Black Tea	1,372
Salada Green Tea—Earl Green	1,250
Lipton Green Tea	1,239
Twinings English Breakfast Tea	935

Adapted from Henning, S. M., Fajardo-Lira, C., Lee, H. W., Youssefian, A. A., Go, V. L., & Heber, D. (2003): Catechin content of 18 teas and a green tea extract supplement correlates with antioxidant capacity. *Nutrition & Cancer*, 45, 226–235. With permission from Lawrence Erlbaum Associates, Inc.

A Glass of Wine and Thou

Wine, particularly red wine, is both a super antioxidant and an NO donor. It offers unique nutritional benefit to sexual vitality as well as cardiovascular and heart health in general.

To ensure sexual vitality and promote vigorous sexual performance after arousal, both men and women must produce NO rapidly and continuously throughout the sexual activity. Red wine has been repeatedly proven to stimulate the production of the endothelial enzyme eNOS, which is required to extract NO from arginine and other food sources (de Gaetano and Cerletti, 2001).

In a recent medical study, eleven healthy nonsmoking men consumed dinner with four glasses of red wine, beer, Dutch gin, or sparkling mineral water (unhappy control group) for three weeks. At the end of the three-week period, serum NO concentrations were measured just before dinner, and one hour, five hours, and thirteen hours after dinner.

Compared with the pre-dinner baseline, both one hour and five hours after dinner, serum NO concentrations were 50 percent higher with any of the alcoholic beverages. After thirteen hours, the NO concentrations returned to baseline levels (Sierksma, van der Gaag, et al., 2003).

Numerous other medical reports conclusively confirm that red wine polyphenols increase endothelial NO release (Leikert, Rathel, et al., 2002). In fact, the polyphenol substances in red wine that increase NO production by the endothelium are now so well known that the term *RWPC*, for "red wine polyphenolic compounds," has entered the scientific vocabulary (Stoclet, Kleschyov, et al., 1999).

RWPCs are known to be beneficial because they can:

- Protect the heart by increasing the good high-density lipoprotein cholesterol (HDL-C), (Rayo Llerena and Marin Huerta, 1998).

- Increase antioxidant activity, thus protecting the endothelium from free radical damage (Hung, Chen, et al., 2000).

- Inhibit the platelet aggregation that can form blood clots and decrease endothelial adhesion so that blood platelets are less likely to cling to the lining of blood vessels and form clots (Bhat, Kosmeder, and Pessuto, 2001; Pignatelli, Pulcinelli, et al., 2000). It will come as no surprise to anyone that a research laboratory located in Bordeaux considers Armagnac the best means of inhibiting platelet aggregation (Umar, Guerin, et al., 2003).

- Prevent accelerated aging of brain cells due to the action of free radicals (Bastianetto and Quirion, 2002).

- Promote the nitric oxide production essential to sexual vitality (Wallerath, Deckert, et al., 2002) while enhancing blood circulation and host immune function (Das, Sato, et al., 1999).

The French Paradox: A Votre Santé

In 1991, the French epidemiologist Serge Renaud outlined on *60 Minutes* his newly minted theory that consuming two to three glasses of wine a day is good for the heart and may forestall death from other causes as well. That TV segment popularized the term *French Paradox* and set off a California wine boom that may have rivaled the Forty-niners' gold rush.

In October 1997, the Novartis Foundation, a prestigious scientific and educational institution founded by the Swiss pharmaceutical company CIBA (now Novartis), held a Symposium on Alcohol and Cardiovascular Diseases in London at which Dr. Renaud presented "The French Paradox and Wine Drinking" (Renaud and Gueguen, 1998).

Dr. Renaud—who to no one's surprise hails from the University of Bordeaux—reported that fewer French die from cardiovascular and heart diseases than do comparable people in any other Western industrialized nation. In fact, they have a 36 percent lower death rate from coronary heart disease (CHD) than Americans, even though their overall mortality rate is only 8 percent lower than ours.

What actually is the "French Paradox"? A study of thirty-four thousand middle-aged French people that spanned twelve years concluded that their average consumption of about 48 g wine per day may be what's responsible for lowering their death rate from cardiovascular disease by 30 or more percent. This helps explain the significantly lower incidence of fatal heart attacks and strokes compared with US rates, despite a "typical French" diet enriched by butter, cream, and high-fat meats (Brouillard, George, and Fougerousse, 1997).

With all our national preoccupation with low-fat, low-cholesterol, and

TABLE 6.4
ORAC Values for Wines

	Alcohol: Actual %	Alcohol: Labeled	Sugar: %	Sulfites: ppm.	Polyphenols: mg/gram	Catechins: mg/175g	Resveratrol: mg/liter
RED WINES							
Rodney Strong Cabernet	10.5	13.8	0	140	3.76	77.3	1.19
Beringer Founders Cabernet	10.5	13.3	0	198	3.62	83.6	0.39
BV Coastal Cabernet	10.5	13	0	122	3.40	69.5	0.43
Yellow Tail Merlot	11.1	13.5	0.5	103	3.26	102.4	2.00
Clos du Bois Merlot	10.8	13	0	140	3.24	93.1	2.28
Rosemount Shiraz	10.9	14	0.2	104	3.22	84.7	2.01
Columbia Crest Merlot/Cab	10.8	13	0	99	3.20	93.6	0.60
Blackstone Merlot	10.7	13	0.4	152	3.05	116.9	1.11
Concha y Toro Merlot	10.3	13	0.4	231	2.77	78.4	5.95
WHITE WINES							
Lindemans Bin 65 Chard	10.7	13.5	0.3	241	0.52	58.9	0.34
Kendall Jackson VR Chard	11.0	13.5	0.6	201	0.48	26.4	0.22
Duboeuf Francais Blanc	10.4	12	0	287	0.47	28.5	0.29
Sutter Home Chardonnay	10.0	13	0.9	205	0.42	36.1	0.09
Woodbridge Chardonnay	11.2	13.5	0	224	0.41	58.3	0.14

	Alcohol: Actual %	Alcohol: Lableled	Sugar: %	Sulfites: ppm.	Polyphenols: mg/gram	Catechins: mg/175g	Resveratrol: mg/liter
Ch. St. Michelle Chardonnay	10.8	13	0.1	208	0.40	39.5	0.09
Fetzer Chardonnay	11.1	13.5	0.4	184	0.39	39.8	0.11
Vendange Chardonnay	10.7	13	0.6	215	0.39	34.6	0.29
Corbett Canyon Chardonnay	10.7	13	0.6	174	0.36	27.9	0.09
Cavit Pinot Grigio	9.6	12	0.4	276	0.35	14.4	0.09
Franzia Chablis (5L box)	8.8	11	1.1	212	0.35	10.2	0.09
Bella Serra Pinot Grigio	9.7	12	0.3	308	0.34	13.5	1.66
Almaden Mt. Chablis	9.4	11.5	0.8	233	0.33	7.3	0.09
Livingston Cellars Chablis	8.4	10.5	1.1	240	0.33	10.7	0.09
Carlo Rossi Chablis	8.2	10.5	1.6	172	0.32	15.2	0.09
Glen Ellen Chardonnay	10.6	13	0.5	154	0.30	27.9	0.09
Bolla Soave	9.7	12	0.2	199	0.30	9.8	0.16
E & J Gallo Chardonnay	10.6	13.5	0.7	153	0.27	15.4	0.09

Adapted from: www.burgundy-talent.com.

low-carb food regimes, what are we doing wrong? Leaving wine off the table may be part of the problem.

The best-known effect of wine and other alcoholic beverages is that they increase circulating serum levels of the good high-density lipoprotein cholesterol. One to two drinks per day increase HDL-C by about 12 percent on average (Linn, Carroll, et al., 1993). This increase is similar to that seen with several other interventions, including exercise programs (Belalcazar and Ballantyne, 1998) and medications.

On the downside, alcohol, like any other source of carbohydrates, can increase plasma triglyceride levels and can serve as a source of excess calories. In individuals with underlying elevated triglycerides, the elevations can be marked (Feinman and Lieber, 1999; Ginsberg, Olefsky, et al., 1974) and have been connected with pancreatic disease.

A recent American Heart Association (AHA)/American College of Cardiology (ACC) consensus panel titled "Guide to Preventive Cardiology for Women" cautioned that women should consume no more than one glass of alcohol per day, because there is some concern that more than 50 g may increase the risk of breast cancer (Mosca, Grundy, et al., 1999). We suggest, whenever possible, that it be one glass of good red wine.

The protective effect of wine seems to depend on whether or not the wine is taken with meals (Criqui, 1998). This may be because the *pattern* of consuming alcoholic beverages can be a marker for other lifestyle factors related to CHD risk (Kauhanen, Kaplan, et al., 1999).

Also, comparing American with European consumers of alcoholic beverages leaves out other important dietary factors such as quantity of fish, fresh fruits, fresh vegetables, and milk consumed. Important risk factors for the incidence of CHD differ not only between Americans and Europeans but also among European subpopulations (Artaud-Wild, Connor, et al., 1993; de Lorgeril, Salen, et al., 1999).

Dr. Denis Blache of the Wine and Vine Institute and Dr. Roger Bessis from the National Institute for Health and Medical Research contend that resveratrol is best obtained by enjoying wine moderately on a routine basis, rather than periodic binge drinking (www.burgundy-talent.com/compnew/english/health/resveratrol.htm).

Like green tea, wine (and other alcoholic beverages) reduces the risk of thrombosis (Klatsky, 1996). Polyphenol antioxidants in red wine neutralize the effects of the disruption in the electrical charge that makes blood platelets aggregate, and also prevent their sticking to vessel walls. There is some evidence that resveratrol and other polyphenolic compounds found especially in red wine can have an independent and additive effect on the reduction of platelet aggregations (Demrow, Slane, and Folts, 1995; Renaud and de Lorgeril, 1992).

The *Cornell Chronicle* reported that New York State wines contain more resveratrol than comparable wines from any other region of the world! Who should know better than Leroy Creasy, the "professor of fruit and vegetable science" (www.news.cornell.edu/Chronicle/98/2.5.98/resveratrol. html)?

Professor Creasy compared many 1995 vintage wines from New York State, California, and other states and countries. Pinot Noir yielded the highest resveratrol content. But Creasy cautioned that each year brings different concentrations, making it difficult for consumers to target the wine best suited to cardiovascular health. Nearly all dark red wines, including Merlot, Cabernet, Zinfandel, Shiraz, and Pinot Noir, contain resveratrol.

We don't advise four glasses of wine with dinner; as Macduff said in the second act of *Macbeth*, ". . . it provokes and unprovokes; it provokes the desire, but it takes away the performance." For many people, a single glass of wine with dinner promotes relaxation and enhances the meal. And it could be that only the cork in the wine bottle separates us from the fountain of cardiovascular youth.

If you avoid alcohol, the good news is that similar antioxidant effects can be obtained from red grape juice (Freedman, Parker, et al., 2001). In fact, it is little known that the antioxidant capacity in red grape juice is superior to that in red wine (Bitsch, Netzel, et al., 2004). A number of websites offer red grape concentrate—even from superior grapes such as Pinot Noir. A few tablespoons in water or seltzer should make a refreshing and healthful beverage.

The American Heart Association maintains its recommendation that alcohol use should be an item of discussion between physician and patient. They also remind us that alcohol is an addictive substance, and adverse effects of drinking occur at more moderate levels in some individuals. It is true that a person's risk for developing alcoholism is difficult, if not impossible, to determine.

A standard drink in the United States is defined as:

- One 12-ounce bottle of domestic-brand popular beer or wine cooler.

- One 5-ounce glass of unfortified table wine or one 2-ounce glass of fortified wine.

- One 1.5-ounce glass of 80-proof distilled spirits (a large shot).

- One 4-ounce glass of liqueur.

Olive Oil: A Legendary Substance

According to Greek mythology, Poseidon, god of the sea, and Athena, goddess of peace and wisdom, held a contest to name a new city in the land of Attica. The prize would be to have the city named after the god who offered the most precious gift to the citizens of the city. When Poseidon struck his trident on a rock, salt flowed forth. Athena upstaged him by striking her spear on the ground and producing an olive tree. Because the olive tree not only lived for hundreds of years, but also gave edible fruits and was the source of oil that could be used to prepare and season food, used as medicine, and used as energy to light their homes, Athena won the contest. The new city was named Athens.

The olive branch remains a symbol of peace, and, fittingly, is the crown given to champions of Olympic sports. As you will see, the respect for the olive tree and its products is well deserved.

Not Less Fat, Better Fat

Recent medical research continues to enhance the legendary status of olive oil. According to a 1997 report in the *New England Journal of Medicine,* women who replaced 5 percent of total daily saturated fat calories with the healthier monounsaturated fat in olive oil were shown to reduce their risk of heart disease by 42 percent (Hu, Stampfer, et al., 1997). This study from the Harvard School of Public Health noted that replacing one type of fat with another is actually more effective in preventing coronary heart disease than is reducing overall fat intake.

Olive oil is, thus, not simply food to the peoples of the Mediterranean region and biblical lands. It is magical, medicinal, and more. The olive tree represents abundance, and its branches, sometimes twisted into a crown, are symbolic of glory, victory, and peace. To this day, the olive branch and the dove symbolize peace and reconciliation in the emblem of the United Nations.

In *The Lexus and the Olive Tree* (2000), the noted *New York Times* columnist Thomas L. Friedman wrote about the emerging world conflict over desire for the products of technology as represented by the Lexus, a luxury, high-tech-assembly-line-produced Japanese automobile, and regional traditions and interests symbolized by the olive tree.

Many of us living in highly developed countries are beginning to look wistfully at simpler, healthier nutrition patterns—those very patterns that evolved over many centuries into traditional regional cuisines. However, due to increasing regional affluence, traditional food choices of Mediterranean populations are rapidly giving way to processed food—especially among the young. In fact, a recent article published by the Department of Pediatrics of the University of Naples asked, "Is the Mediterranean Diet Becoming Obsolete?" (Greco, Musmarra, et al., 1998).

Here is a curious paradox: Populations that inherited a culture of healthy nutrition seem to be "evolving" toward exchanging those foods for the unhealthy foods of the Western world. This is happening just as food scientists in the Western world are touting the benefits of a simpler diet.

Most recently, investigators from the Institute of Cardiovascular Disease, Department of Pathology, University of California, San Francisco, examined nine thousand men and women from six different regions of Turkey. Turkey seems an ideal laboratory for such a study since its various geographic regions differ markedly in diet, ranging from the Aegean coast diet high in olive oil to an Anatolian diet emphasizing meat and dairy products.

The rural population consuming an olive-oil-rich diet had the lowest plasma cholesterol (hovering around 149 mg/dl for both men and women). The urban population of Istanbul and Adana had higher levels (ranging in men and women from 292 to 184 mg/dl). Affluent men had the highest cholesterol levels—207 mg/dl (Mahley, Palaoglu, et al., 1995).

Affluence and higher education were associated with higher cholesterol levels, as were lack of physical activity, smoking, and alcohol consumption. Where nutrition is concerned, affluence does not necessarily translate to better health.

SAD

Health authorities have created a depressing new acronym: *SAD*, standing for "standard American diet." It is a fitting term because, as we have seen, our typical diet is painfully deficient in core nutrients. Most importantly, as regards sexual function, our national diet fails to provide the powerful NO fuel and antioxidants to support sexual performance. Right now, our national daily intake provides about 35 percent of its calories in the form of sugar and 45 percent in the form of fat. Thirty-three percent of Americans are niacin-deficient, 34 percent are deficient in vitamin B_{12}, 34 percent are deficient in riboflavin, 41 percent in vitamin C, 45 percent in thiamine, 50 percent in vitamin A, 50 percent in iron, 68 percent in calcium, 75 percent in magnesium, and 90 in vitamin B_6 (www.renewalresearch.com).

How can olive oil help us improve our statistics? We discussed the French Paradox regarding wine. Consider the Albanian Paradox. Albania is generally regarded as the poorest country in Europe. But the death rate attributable to coronary heart disease in adult Albanian men is less than half the rate found in the United States. Similar to what is seen in Italy, mortality is lowest in southwestern Albania—where most of that country's fruits and vegetables are grown and consumed, and where most of the olive oil is produced and consumed. This is a living example of the benefits of the Mediterranean diet, where olive products are a staple in every household.

In general, lower mortality rates are seen in regions of the Mediterranean where the diet is consistently low in consumption of total calories per day, meat, and milk products, and where there is high consumption of fruits, vegetables, carbohydrates, and olive oil (Gjonka and Bobak, 1998). This leads us to speculate that perhaps the olive is the nutritional secret of generations of Latin lovers.

A Brief History of Olive Cultivation and Use

The olive tree and its fruit (the drupe), leaves, and wood have featured prominently in the history of the Greater Mediterranean. Olive cultivation is thought to have originated in what is now Syria, from where olive trees spread all over the world. Olives appear in what may be the oldest known cookbook, the two-thousand-year-old Roman *De re Coquinaria* (www.earthy.com/goto.htm).

Today olives are commercially exploited throughout the Mediterranean, especially Greece and Spain. They are also prominent in the economies of New Zealand, South Africa, and California.

Franciscan missionaries planted the first olive trees in California around 1769 (www.soupsong.com). These evergreen trees can grow to heights from 20 to 40 feet and live to a prodigious age. It is estimated that some in the eastern Mediterranean region may be well over two thousand years old. Somewhere between the ages of four and five, they begin to bear fruit.

It is estimated that there are about eight hundred million olive trees growing in the world at this time, everywhere from Spain, Italy, France, Greece, Tunisia, Morocco, Turkey, Portugal, China, Chile, Peru, Brazil, Mexico, Angola, South Africa, Uruguay, Afghanistan, and Australia to the United States (www.theolivepress.com).

When taken directly off the branches of the tree, olives are not very tasty because of the acrid oleuropin in their skin. This substance does not affect the production of oil, though it is removed when the olives are intended for table use. There are several common methods of "curing" olives: several months of soaking in oil, in water, or in brine; or dry-curing by packing in salt or an alkaline medium such as lye.

What Does the Label Tell Us About the Oil?

First, the quality of olive oil is judged chemically to determine its acidity. The highest-quality olive oil has the lowest acidity level: Extra-virgin olive oil has an acidity level of less than 1 percent, or 1 g per 100 g of oil. Additionally, extra-virgin olive oil must meet certain aroma, flavor, and color criteria that are subjectively established by a panel of expert judges.

Virgin olive oil, by contrast, must have an acidity level that does not exceed 1.5 percent while at the same time meeting the same aroma, flavor, and color criteria as its extra-virgin counterpart.

Ordinary olive oil is virgin olive oil with an acidity level of less than 3.3 percent. Olive oil with an acidity level greater than 3.3 percent is considered unsuitable for human consumption as food and it is usually put to other commercial uses.

Pure olive oil is a low-cost blend of refined and virgin olive oil. Researchers from a medical unit investigating cardiovascular epidemiology in

Barcelona, Spain, found that extra-virgin olive oil contains phenolic compounds that protect LDL cholesterol from free-radical oxidation better than refined oil without such phenolic compounds (Fito, Covas, et al., 2000).

Olive oil does not require refrigeration but should be kept in a dark, cool place. Buy it in glass bottles rather than plastic, because it can absorb some of the components of plastic. Its shelf life is about two years; after that, it should be discarded.

It is easy to make olive oil the oil of choice for your kitchen. Just substitute it for any other cooking and/or salad oil. To keep calories down, olive oil can be sprayed onto cooking surfaces, rather than poured, by using a spray bottle.

- **Olive oil,** 1 tablespoon: 119 calories, 13.5 g total fat.

Not Just for Martinis

Adding whole olives to your plate is another way to reap the benefits of their powerful antioxidant effects. Olives come in a wide variety of colors, reflecting their stage of ripeness. Raw green olives are the youngest; they turn purplish red and finally black as they mature. Fresh olives are soaked (often in a solution containing lye) to remove the bitter taste and then cured in brine (salt water) or in oil. They may finally be packed in oil, vinegar, herbs, or spices (www.soupsong.com). The typical olive has about 15 calories, due to the high fat content in the form of oil.

Try adding olives to salads, or blending olives and cottage cheese as a light spread. Olives are also delicious when added to fish dishes.

- **Olives,** pickled, canned or bottled, green, 100 g: 145 calories, 15.3 g total fat, 1,556 mg sodium.

- **Olives,** ripe, canned, any size, 100 g: 115 calories, 10.7 g total fat, 872 mg sodium.

Grape Seed Extract (Oil)

Sexual vitality depends principally on the production of nitric oxide locally in the sex organs at the instigation of erotic desire. Therefore, nutrients that increase NO production promote increased blood flow to those organs requiring arousal: erection of the penis in men, and labial and clitoral engorgement and lubrication in women.

In some cases, foods such as those high in nitrates and arginine contribute directly to what's needed to supply NO. In other cases, just as important but indirectly, foods prevent hazards to vigorous sexual function such as free radical damage to the endothelium, high blood pressure, and high serum LDL cholesterol. In many cases, as you have seen, foods perform more than one beneficial function—for example, dietary olive oil as salad dressing or for cooking.

Another highly beneficial oil is made from grape seed extract. Grape seed extract is derived from the seeds of red wine grapes. The oil is rich in proanthocyanidins, among the most powerful antioxidants that nature provides.

Many recent studies show conclusively that grape seed extract, especially the one that medical scientists now identify as IH636 grape seed proanthocyanidin extract (GSPE), is one of the most powerful and effective antioxidants known (Bagchi, Bagchi, et al., 2000). Proanthocyanidins in grape seed oil protect the endothelium from free radical damage (Bagchi, Bagchi, et al., 2002) and enhance the action of NO (Aldini, Carini, et al., 2003).

An enzyme in human female breast tissue converts androgen into estrogen. This enzyme is significantly more active in breast cancer tissue than in comparable noncancerous tissue. A fraction from grape seed oil (and red wine as well) inhibits the elevated expression of that enzyme (Eng, Ye, et al., 2003). In another study, a treatment combination including grape seed oil enhanced the effectiveness of chemotherapy for treatment of breast carcinoma (Sharma, Tyagi, et al., 2004). Grape seed extract (oil) inhibited tumor growth by 60 to 70 percent when human prostate cancer was implanted in laboratory mice. The researchers proposed including it in treatment of cancer in human patients (Singh, Tyagi, et al., 2004).

One grape seed fraction is an ACE (angiotensin-converting enzyme) inhibitor (Uchida, Ikari, et al., 1987). Drugs inhibiting the action of this enzyme help lower blood pressure by regulating sodium and water retention in patients with essential hypertension, a hazard to sexual vitality.

The most valuable flavonoids in grape seed extract are procyanidolic oligomers—also known as proanthocyanidins but commonly called

OPCs. Physicians in Europe now commonly prescribe proanthocyanidin-containing drugs for various blood vessel disorders and for diabetes, leg cramps, varicose veins, arm and leg numbness or tingling, age-related macular degeneration, and even impotence. Grape seed extract can block prostaglandins and therefore may reduce the severity of endometriosis.

Grape seed oil has a relatively high smoke point, approximately 320 degrees Fahrenheit, so it can be safely used to cook at high temperatures. It can be used for stir-fries, sautéing, and fondue. It is prized for its clean, light taste, making it a good choice for salad dressing as well as cooking delicate white fish. Because of its neutral taste, grape seed oil makes a great base for infusing or flavoring with garlic, rosemary, or other herbs or spices.

- **Grape seed oil,** 1 cup: zero protein, no value known for arginine, 1,927 calories, 218 g total fat, zero cholesterol and sodium.

Beyond Food

Beauty and the Grape Seed

Supermodel Carla Bruni and Princess Caroline of Monaco reportedly use one of the most effective anti-aging, anti-wrinkle creams available today: Lait Corporel eau Pépins de Raisins (body lotion from grape seeds), made by Caudalie Cosmetics. The key ingredient is grape seed extract, which, barring allergic reaction, can be applied directly to the face. Proanthocyanidins protect the skin from free radical damage caused by exposure to ultraviolet sun radiation and can even repair some of that damage. Other beauty manufacturers are catching on—Lancôme's Vinefit also contains grape seed oil.

"Of Mice and Men"—Gone Today . . . Hair Tomorrow?

In 1998, scientists from a well-known and respected Japanese laboratory reported their discovery that grape seed proanthocyanidin extract promotes hair growth. They tested their discovery by observing its hair-growth-promoting activity in isolated mouse hair follicles in laboratory dish preparations (in vitro).

They observed the same phenomenon in tests on live bald mice (in vivo). Not surprisingly, the active fractions that they isolated from grape seed extract were the same as those found in red wine (Takahashi, Kamyia, and Yokoo, 1998). GSPE was also found to be superior to minoxidil in growth-promoting activity. They proposed GSPE as an active agent for curing androgenic alopecia—male pattern baldness.

The following year, they reported in the *Journal of Investigative Dermatology* that they had further evidence of the active growth-promoting substance in GSPE and again recommended it for potential use as an agent to induce hair growth (Takahashi, Kamyia, et al., 1999). Human pilot and toxicological studies were conducted in 1999, and showed that their substance, procyanidin B_2, is safe for topical use and effective in curing androgenic alopecia (Takahashi, Yokoo, et al., 1999).

Massage and Lubrication

Because of its light texture and ability to form a moisture-retaining film, grape seed oil is also excellent as massage oil. It can also be used as a natural lubricant to counter vaginal dryness and improve sexual enjoyment. Be sure to do a "patch test" first on a small area of skin (such as the underside of your arm) to make sure you are not allergic to it.

Chocolate

> *Chocolate is a perfect food, as wholesome as it is delicious, a beneficent restorer of exhausted power.*
> —BARON JUSTUS VON LIEBIG (1803–1873), German chemist

Chocolate lovers of the world, rejoice! Medical science keeps identifying more and more reasons to eat (a reasonable amount of) this delicious substance on a regular basis. And we do consume chocolate at an incredible rate: Recent data released in a report by the business information group Datamonitor revealed that the global consumption of chocolate totaled approximately $42.2 billion annually (www.datamonitor.com/~2bbf82da 36b94b5aa3c760fbee2ea5e0~/all/news/product.asp?pid=0033901A-F384-4A0B-A5A9-AF0D14901DF1).

Chocolate is a well-established symbol of romance and the gift of choice worldwide on Valentine's Day. It turns out that chocolate is an excellent choice for the day dedicated to love, because it's a powerful stimulant that enhances the nitric oxide formation needed for vigorous love-making (Karim, McCormick, and Kappagoda, 2000).

Chocolate Sources

Chocolate is made from the seeds of the cacao tree. It was enjoyed in the prehistoric societies of Central American and later in Mayan and Aztec civilizations. It played an important part in religious, medical, economic, and social history around the world.

Chocolate has been credited as an aphrodisiac and an antidepressant. Cacao beans were so highly valued that they were used as currency in Mesoamerica and only turned into food after becoming too worn to trade.

In 1828, Dutch chocolate maker Conrad J. van Houten patented an inexpensive method for pressing the fat from roasted cacao beans; he also created cocoa powder. This paved the way for the production of chocolate bars. Hershey mass-marketed the first bar in 1900, and US production soared during World War II, when chocolate bars were put into the pockets of soldiers as they were sent off to war.

Delicious Nutrition

Chocolate has an exceptionally high ORAC value—one of the highest among antioxidants. There are 6,560 ORAC units in a 50-g serving of dark chocolate, versus 455 units in a 50-g serving of broccoli, making chocolate fourteen and a half times more powerful an antioxidant. Could this be why a bouquet of broccoli never caught on for Valentine's Day?

Chocolate is healthy for your love life in more ways than one: Flavonoids in cocoa protect against coronary heart disease because they promote the NO that keeps blood flowing freely to the heart (Fisher, Hughes, et al., 2003). They also inhibit LDL-C oxidation, thus forestalling atherosclerosis (Mathur, Devaraj, et al., 2002). As noted earlier, when above-the-waist organs benefit, so do their below-the-waist counterparts.

Dark chocolate has received recent attention for its positive effect on high blood pressure. Dark chocolate is rich in flavonoids due to its high cocoa content. Writing in the journal *Hypertension*, Dr. David Grassi, from the University of L'Aquila in Italy, and colleagues describe studies done with a high-flavonol preparation of dark chocolate that has been shown to decrease blood pressure and insulin resistance in healthy volunteers as well as patients with clinically documented high blood pressure. These trials were probably notable for how easy it was to recruit participants!

How do cocoa flavonoids and other polyphenolic compounds stack up against other super antioxidants? Writing in the *Journal of Agricultural & Food Chemistry*, scientists compared cocoa with other antioxidants using a very sophisticated chemical analysis. Here's what they found for comparable servings:

- Cocoa has 611 mg phenols and 564 mg flavonoids.
- Red wine has 340 mg phenols and 163 mg flavonoids.
- Green tea has 165 mg phenols and 47 mg flavonoids.
- Black tea has 124 mg phenols and 34 mg flavonoids.

Clearly, cocoa has a greater antioxidant capacity per serving than either tea or wine (Lee, Kim, and Lee, 2003). What's more, the epicatechin antioxidant in cocoa is rapidly bioavailable to begin mopping up free radicals—within two hours (Wang, Schramm, et al., 2000). And NO production is dose-dependent: The more flavonoids there are in the cocoa, the more NO is produced in the body. Scientists at Mars Inc., the candy company, even calculated the ORAC equivalent of concentrations of procyanins in cocoa (Adamson, Lazarus, et al., 1999).

Chocolate comes in all shapes and forms, including powder, bars, chips, and chunks. It also varies in sweetness, depending on the amount of sugar added, and creaminess, depending on the amount of cocoa butter added. The "chocolatiness" depends on the concentration of the chocolate "liquor" to other ingredients such as milk or sugar.

Different types of chocolate contain different amounts of theobromine, the main active stimulant in cocoa. In general, theobromine levels are higher in dark chocolate (approximately 10 g per kg) than in milk chocolate (1 to 5 g per kg). Higher-quality chocolate tends to contain more theobromine than lower-quality chocolate. Cocoa beans are naturally variable in theobromine content, ranging from approximately 300 to 1,200 mg per ounce.

We have two important cautions about chocolate, however. First, no matter how much you love your dog, don't feed it chocolate: Cocoa and chocolate products may be toxic, even lethal, to dogs. Theobromine adversely affects their heart, central nervous system, and kidneys.

Also, if you're prone to migraine headaches, it is important not to overindulge in chocolate. Depending on your sensitivity, even small amounts have been reported to trigger headaches. That will certainly put a damper on any plans for sex.

These caveats aside: Put a chocolate kiss on the pillow and get into bed!

• **Dark chocolate, bar,** 1.45-ounce (41-g) serving: 2 g protein, no value known for arginine, 218 calories, 13 g total fat, 2 mg cholesterol, 2 mg sodium.

• **Milk chocolate, chips,** 1-cup (168-g, 6-ounce) serving : 13 g protein, 501 mg arginine, 899 calories, 50 g total fat, 39 mg cholesterol, 133 mg sodium.

7

A Simple Nutritional Plan for a Lifetime of Healthy Sex

From the Kitchen to the Bedroom

It's time to get down to the basics of eating. Great food and great sex both depend on one thing—variety. And variety is the main ingredient in our Great Food, Great Sex eating plan as well.

Every Great Food, Great Sex plate offers up foods rich in vibrant color and interesting texture. Our plan encourages consumption of a wide range of foods while avoiding overconsumption of any one type. This is the key to a healthy, balanced food plan that you can use for the rest of your life, as well as for every member of your family. Why do we say that? Because the Great Food, Great Sex plan is first and foremost a heart-healthy nutrition plan, based on the core concept of a unified circulatory system. What is good for you above the belt is great for you below the belt.

Planning your meals, as well as those of your loved ones, according to the simple, easy-to-implement Food Factor principles ensures that every meal you prepare will be full of great nutrition and low in saturated fat and refined sugar.

Think of your plate as a palette of beautiful colors. Try to arrange your meals so that rich green, red, yellow, and/or orange foods are highly visible. Pick red cabbage over white, sweet potatoes over french fries, and mesclun greens over iceberg lettuce.

Find places for tomatoes and squash. Practice food presentation as if you were dining in a fine restaurant and using colored foods for garnish as well as portion. Let your imagination run wild, and try to think of a dessert that uses more than one type of fruit—think berries, mangoes, pineapple, kiwi, pomegranate, *and* grapes.

HUNGER VERSUS APPETITE

Like all living creatures, we are endowed with a hunger drive. Our brain has a hunger control system often mislabeled the appetite control system (ACS). This system integrates information about body weight, activity level, hormone status, and so on to regulate food intake. If we do not satisfy hunger, we can damage our body. We are also endowed with an appetitive drive. If we do not satisfy it, we may experience discomfort, but it will not result in harm.

Culinary customs, often cultural phenomena, typically contrive to combine hunger and appetite in food preparation so as to reduce hunger and, at the same time, increase appetite. Appetite for certain foods and tastes is part of the cement that binds us to our cultures. Thus, food preparation may create an appetitive drive to which all sorts of nonfood stimuli and symbols are attached: We do not consume ice cream for its calcium content, we do not eat sushi to obtain omega-3 fish oil, and we do not eat pizza for the lycopene in the tomato sauce.

It can be difficult to alter ingrained habits when it comes to food. This is in part because we fear withdrawal from foods that we crave, even when we can satisfy hunger with many other more nutritious choices. Think about it: We can satisfy hunger more easily than we can satisfy appetite. Here is an example: A woman being treated for migraine headaches began keeping a food log in addition to a symptom log. After a week or so, she realized that her migraines seemed to be most common on days when she consumed foods high in wheat. When her doctor suggested that she try to avoid high-wheat foods, however, she shot back, "But there's nothing else to eat!" This knee-jerk reaction is a typical response to diets with significant food restrictions.

Have no fear—the advantage of our diet is that it promotes health without triggering the hunger–appetite conflict. We encourage you to look through the various food lists and pick out your favorites in each group. All the foods in our plan are common. In addition, try experimenting with fruits and vegetables that are new to you. Like trying a new position for sex, you may be pleasantly surprised by the experience of a new flavor or texture.

There are almost endless combinations of food that can be eaten to achieve high ORAC and high NO levels in nutrition. We have ranked the most common foods in accordance with their nitrogen compound NO-donor value, their arginine NO-donor value, and their antioxidant value. You can also easily calculate values for any foods not included in our lists by using one of the many nutrition websites available on the Internet. Try www.wholehealthmd.com or www.nutritiondata.com.

EASY DOES IT

The Great Food, Great Sex plan is one of the few diet plans around that does not require you to become an expert in nutrition. Our food plan has no known hazards because it is based on a sane combination of commonly eaten foods. These foods are simply ranked in accordance with certain key constituents that, if consumed in combination, add up to zest in the bedroom.

We don't ask you to *restrict* foods as much as *introduce* more foods that are healthy for your entire body. By following the simple guidelines for the three Food Factors, you can plan your meals to be delicious, nutritious, and visually appealing. And the reward for compliance is better and better sex.

If you are like almost half of the American population, you may benefit from weight loss as well. Unlike the constant supply of fad diets, our Great Food, Great Sex plan is based on a wide range of healthy foods and does not create nutritional deficiencies. Even though this program is not primarily designed to promote weight loss, the plan calls for high consumption of fruits, vegetables, and lean fish, meat, and poultry. Combine that with vigorous lovemaking, and weight loss could well become inevitable.

The advantage of basing our plan for sexual vitality on the three Food Factors is that it does not require elimination of any food category from the diet. Therefore, you won't experience withdrawal discomfort. In fact, the plan encourages increasing consumption of some foods and the addition of other foods that are missing from the SAD (standard American diet) eating patterns.

Consider a typical day on the SAD:

Breakfast

- 1 egg scrambled in 1 teaspoon butter.
- 2 slices white toast.
- 1 teaspoon butter.
- ½ cup apple juice.

Snack

- 1 doughnut or piece of cake.

Lunch

- 1 ham-and-cheese sandwich (2 ounces meat, 1 ounce cheese) on white bread.
- 1 teaspoon mayonnaise.
- 3-ounce bag potato chips.
- 12-ounce soft drink.
- 2 chocolate chip cookies.

Snack

- 8 Wheat Thins.

Dinner

- 3 ounces broiled sirloin.
- 1 medium baked potato.
- 1 tablespoon sour cream.
- 1 teaspoon butter.
- ½ cup peas with ½ teaspoon butter.

This is a day of what nutritionists like to refer to as "empty" calories from food that supplies high amounts of sugar and fat. Now consider a typical day on the Great Food, Great Sex plan:

Breakfast

- 1 mushroom and spinach omelet.
- 1 slice whole wheat toast.
- 1 teaspoon apple butter.
- 1 fresh melon wedge.

Snack

- 1 cup fresh strawberries.

Lunch

- 1 tuna sandwich (3.5 ounces of fish, 1 stick celery, ½ chopped apple) on whole wheat pita bread.
- 1 teaspoon mayonnaise.
- Carrot sticks.
- Iced green tea.
- 1 square dark chocolate.

Snack

- ½ cup toasted almonds.

Dinner

- 3 ounces baked pork chop.
- 1 medium baked sweet potato.
- 1 mixed green salad with olive oil and balsamic vinegar.
- ½ cup string beans tossed with seasoned olive oil.
- 1 to 2 glasses red wine.

As you can see, the calories in the Great Food, Great Sex foods are loaded with the nutrients needed for an energetic lifestyle, in the bedroom as well as out of it.

The three Food Factors for sexual vitality are not magical, even though eating this way can transform your sex life. The foods in our plan are very similar to those eaten in many parts of the world and known as the Mediterranean diet. This diet, low in red meat and high in green and yellow vegetables, fruits, fish, olive oil, and nuts—not to mention red wine—has been frequently recommended for its cardiovascular benefits.

One difference is that our plan is not as restrictive in red meat (a high source of arginine), though it balances it with endothelium-protective antioxidants. These benefits translate nicely from the kitchen to the bedroom.

Much of the Mediterranean diet, as we know it today, evolved from regional nutrition practices that probably existed long before Homer wrote the *Odyssey*, lasting through the biblical era and on to the recent past. What did Odysseus share with his wife, Penelope, before setting out on his famous voyage?

Food residues from a burial banquet found in the tomb of King Midas, in western Turkey, that dates back some twenty-seven hundred years give us an idea of the very early Mediterranean diet:

- A Turkish meze of goat cheese, julienned cucumbers, asparagus, arugula, olive and garbanzo spread, dried figs, and a cornelian cherry vinaigrette.
- Spicy lamb and lentil stew.
- A mixture of honey mead, beer, and wine, spiced with saffron.
- A honey and caramelized-fennel dessert tart.

Not a bad send-off. Another source tells us that the following is a sample meal from ancient Greece (www.fjkluth.com/daily.html):

- Flat bread containing barley.
- Shish kebab with lamb (marinated in olive oil and red wine), beans, cabbage, apples, and pears.
- Thyme was a likely herb.
- Baklava for dessert.

These foods are entirely consistent with cardiovascular and heart health as well as sexual vitality. Yet all these dishes were also made from readily available ingredients. There was no Burger King in the Athenian agora, no Big Bob's on Mount Parnassus, no McDonald's across the square from the Temple of Athena. But those benefits are beginning to be lost as the SAD makes its way across the world.

SADDER, NOT WISER

The US Department of Agriculture has reported that fifty-eight thousand metric tons of french fries—$45 million worth—were consumed in restaurants in Greece in 1997 (www.fas.usda.gov). To no one's surprise, as eating patterns change, the Greek incidence of cardiovascular and heart disease and stroke has approached ours (Panagiotakos, Chrysohoou, et al., 2003).

Achilles did not have to decide between soggy Cocoa Puffs with a glass of orange drink (sweetened with high-fructose corn syrup) and goat's-milk yogurt with fresh figs for breakfast. Xanthippe did not face the choice of a peanut butter and jelly sandwich on white bread with a Coke, versus shish kebab with lamb, beans, cabbage, apples, pears, and wine to serve Socrates for lunch before he returned to his afternoon sophistry session behind the agora. Penelope did not weigh a hamburger, french fries, and a chocolate shake against fresh vegetables and a fish fillet—with red wine—for lunch to serve Odysseus before his momentous voyage.

If we want to adopt permanent dietary habits that will keep us healthy, young, and sexy, it is not enough to read about it. We do have to make *some* changes in our eating behavior to achieve our goals.

A GENERAL PRINCIPLE: BROWN IS THE NEW WHITE

The Atkins and son-of-Atkins diets made *carb* the newest four-letter word in our society. This is another example of going overboard with what was originally a reasonable idea. A more sensible approach to carbohydrate consumption, especially for the long term, is to choose a brown food over a white one whenever possible. Examples are whole-grain bread, whole-grain pasta, and brown rice. The brown color in these foods results from their being "whole" rather than "overprocessed" foods; they retain the fiber content of the original ingredients.

White overprocessed foods, made primarily from highly refined flour and sugar, are an insult to your pancreas: These foods can cause a rapid rise in blood sugar followed by a rapid rise in insulin. As the insulin neutralizes the high blood sugar, many people experience a comparably rapid drop in blood sugar, leaving them tired, cranky, and, in many cases, with a headache. These are not conditions likely to lead to satisfying lovemaking. No wonder, "Not tonight, dear. I have a headache."

In addition, these foods can make it easier to gain weight, because whatever highly refined carbohydrate is left in your system after your basic energy needs have been met gets stockpiled as fat for future energy needs. This helps explain why the only people who can eat these foods without worrying about weight gain tend to be competitive athletes whose bodies have very high energy requirements.

For the rest of us, the secret to attaining and maintaining desirable weight (and often the weight at which we will feel most desirable) is modest portions of carbohydrates that are closer to the way they were created in nature—brown, not white.

We gratefully acknowledge the contribution of many of our recipes from programs developed by the National Heart, Lung, and Blood Institute (NHLBI) of the National Institutes of Health (NIH). Our government is funding research to actively investigate the nutritional benefits of NO in the treatment of patients with heart disease.

We extend that science to the table and bedroom of the general population. Our dietary recommendations, with the help of these NIH-sponsored clinical trials, are scientifically and nutritionally sound. We believe that with proper care and feeding, you can stay healthy over many years of vigorous and joyful lovemaking.

GET READY TO X-RATE YOUR PLATE

Our plan is remarkably easy to implement using the three Food Factors as the basis for food selection and meal planning. Promoting permanent change is best done in stages. Because our national diet is already high in protein, we encourage moving toward leaner forms of protein, as well as including more fish.

For many people, increasing daily consumption of fruits and vegetables may be more challenging. This is a lifetime food plan, so allow yourself time to adapt to a different style of eating. The Great Food, Great Sex plan is designed to provide a nutritionally complete and sensible balance of reduced-fat, high-protein foods with endothelium-preserving antioxidant foods.

The core nutritional guidelines are listed below.

A Daily Nutritional Arginine Intake of 2,500 to 3,500 Milligrams

For example, 3.5 ounces of white-meat chicken, a normal portion for dinner, supplies almost 1,400 mg arginine. Add to this a handful of nuts (732 mg per ounce) for a snack and a tuna salad (1,413 mg) and you are over the top. This is an easy goal because you have many choices from two Food Factor groups.

- If you traditionally eat little protein, gradually add Greens and Beans and Staminators to reach your goal over several weeks. Greens and Beans will be the mainstay for arginine intake if you follow a vegetarian diet.
- Try to eat foods from both groups.
- Try to have beans at least three times a week—they supply fiber as well as arginine. Beans can be added to soups, stews, and salads as well as any rice dish.

A Daily ORAC Intake of at Least 5,000 Units

If your current idea of fruits and vegetables is a glass of frozen orange juice for breakfast and the pickle with your hamburger, you are in for a lot of fun. The Brights add color, texture, and zest to your meals while protecting your endothelium for great sexual function.

Many of us learned to dislike vegetables by only tasting them when they were served overcooked and uninspired. A large salad for lunch and/or dinner is a great way to combine both raw and cooked vegetables. Experiment by adding fresh herbs and spices to olive oil to make tasty dressings.

The goal is to gradually add fresh fruits and vegetables into your daily menu until you are eating seven to ten servings per day. One serving is, for example, ½ cup berries, 1 sweet potato, or a cup of cooked green beans.

- Choose fruits with high ORAC values whenever possible.

- Choose brightly colored vegetables whenever possible, including deep green vegetables.

- When eating out, ask for a second green vegetable in place of potatoes or rice.

- Snack on cherry tomatoes, celery, and baby carrots for a low-cal pick-me-up.

- Fruit is not just for breakfast: Get in the habit of using fresh fruit as a midmorning and/or afternoon snack to maintain even blood sugar levels.

- Experiment with a wide range of fruits.

- Have fresh berries whenever possible, but use fresh-frozen if they're easier to obtain.

- Try keeping a bowl of fruit in the refrigerator to tempt you for a tasty snack.

- Get in the habit of bringing fruit to work as an alternative to the 3:00 P.M. potato chip break.

- Purée fruits like peaches and berries in the blender and use as a sauce over melons.

Eat Fish at Least Twice a Week

- Fish can be eaten at any meal—try smoked salmon for breakfast.

- Fish can be prepared whole, as fillets, or in soups, stews, or casseroles.

- Experiment with different types of fish to find the ones you enjoy most.

Enjoy a Handful of Raw or Roasted Nuts or a Tablespoon of Nut Butter Every Day

- Nuts make a great midafternoon snack in place of chips or cookies.

- Add nuts to salads for a satisfying crunch.

Keep Cholesterol in Check

- When making omelets, use three egg whites and one yolk per omelet.
- Select lean meats whenever possible.
- Pour off fat when pan-broiling meat.

Drink Green Tea

- Try to have at least one serving of green tea every day.
- Whenever possible, drink green tea in place of coffee or black tea.
- Try iced green tea instead of soda.
- Visit a Japanese food store or sushi take-out restaurant for a wide variety of green teas.

Use Olive Oil and/or Grape Seed Oil for Cooking, Seasoning, and Salad Dressings

- Instead of butter on your dinner roll, put fresh red pepper and a crushed clove of garlic in a small dish of olive oil and dip crusty Italian bread in the mixture.
- Substitute oil in any recipe calling for margarine.

Enjoy a Glass of Red Wine or Grape Juice with Dinner

- Experiment with a variety of wines.
- Consider going to a wine-tasting course to learn more.
- Ask for recommendations from friends and co-workers.
- If alcohol is in your "no fly zone," use grape juice. It has the same nutritional benefits as wine—in some cases, even more—without the issues.

Stock Your Kitchen with "Sexy Staples"

- Shop for a variety of beans.
- Dry beans require soaking for several hours before cooking. Or you can freeze them in a plastic container of water, then place the frozen block in a pot and cook as usual.

- If you're using canned beans, place them in a strainer and rinse to remove extra salt.

- Add a variety of raw unsalted nuts to your diet. If you don't like the flavor of raw nuts, they can be gently toasted in a baking pan in the oven or in a heavy saucepan on top of the stove. Try adding a teaspoon of tamari soy sauce to the pan for a saltier taste.

- Try serving a variety of olives with raw carrots, peppers, and celery for a tasty appetizer.

- Experiment with a variety of whole olives.

- Consider adding olives to salads, as an appetizer, or in stews.

- You'll need to stock up on olive oil.

- Have available a range of dried fruits: dates, figs, raisins, apricots, and so on.

- Fresh and dried spices can keep things interesting. Basics include cinnamon, nutmeg, ginger, turmeric, hot pepper, and garlic.

Choose Whole-Grain Products Whenever Possible

- Breads, cereal, and rice have a higher nutritional value when made from whole grains.

- The fiber in whole-grain products helps keep blood sugar stable and promotes digestion.

Shop for Fresh Food Whenever Possible

- Fresh food ordering and delivery via the Internet is becoming increasingly popular and available in more neighborhoods.

- Explore ethnic markets for new and interesting fruits, vegetables, and spices.

SALT INTAKE

The minimum daily requirement of sodium in the human diet is 500 mg, about ¼ teaspoon of salt. The typical American diet includes about

6,000 mg of sodium (1 tablespoon salt). The Nutrition Institute recommends 1,000 to 3,000 mg of sodium per day, or about ½ to 1½ teaspoons of salt. That may be far too high. The closer to 1,000, or less, the better.

Here is a list of the sodium content of foods, by groups.

Vegetables and Fruits

- Fresh or frozen vegetables, 35 mg per ½ cup.
- Canned vegetables, 140 to 160 mg per ½ cup.
- Fresh, frozen, canned fruits, 8 mg per ½ cup.

Milk Group

- Milk, 125 mg per 1 cup.
- Cottage cheese, 450 mg per ½ cup.
- Natural cheese (Swiss, cheddar), 125 to 150 mg per ounce.
- Processed cheese (Parmesan), 350 to 450 mg per ounce.

Meat Group

- Fresh meat, poultry, fish, 75 mg per 3.3-ounce (average) serving.
- Cured meat, hot dogs, 750 to 1,000 mg per ounce.
- Eggs, 60 mg each.
- Fats (margarine, butter), 25 to 30 mg per 1 teaspoon or 1 pat butter.
- Grains, cereals, potatoes, 5 mg per ½ cup.

WEIGHT LOSS ON THE GREAT FOOD, GREAT SEX PLAN

Trying to cut calories? Cut your grape juice with seltzer, add a slice of lemon, and you have a delicious, refreshing beverage. Most importantly, make mealtimes pleasurable. Prepare and eat foods you enjoy, and make the extra effort to set an attractive table whenever possible. A successful restaurant usually owes its popularity to its atmosphere as well as its cuisine.

- Whenever possible, eat meals when you are truly hungry, rather than eating by the clock.

- Try leaving several bites of food on your plate at each meal.

- Avoid eating on the run—sit down whenever you eat.

- Stop halfway through each meal and monitor your sense of fullness.

- When eating at a restaurant with large portions, ask for a second plate and have "leftovers" packed up *before* you begin eating.

- Substitute an additional cooked vegetable and/or larger serving of salad for potatoes, pasta, or rice.

- Have a glass of (low-sodium) tomato or vegetable juice before dinner.

- Walk during the day whenever possible.

- Try keeping a simple food diary of what you are eating.

ONE-WEEK SAMPLE PLAN

The Great Food, Great Sex meal plan is as simple or as elaborate as you wish to make it. We have provided examples of a week's worth of meals based on the principles of the three Food Factors, but feel free to experiment with your own food plan.

If you enjoy cooking, try making your own recipes from the three Food Factor foods. We suggest making multiple servings when you cook so that you can use a dinner dish for lunch. Try making soup on a regular basis, and freezing portions for a quick meal.

	Monday	Tuesday	Wednesday	Thursday	Friday	Saturday	Sunday
BREAKFAST	• Good Morning Muesli	• BananaBerry Smoothie • Krisp bread	• Frisky Veggie Frittata • Whole-grain toast	• Seasonal melon with cottage cheese • Melba toast	• Poached eggs on English muffin • Sliced berries	• Mango for It	• Breakfast Burrito
SNACK	• Whole fresh fruit	• Whole fresh fruit	• Whole fresh fruit	• Whole fresh fruit	• Whole fresh fruit	• Whole fresh fruit	• Whole fresh fruit
LUNCH	• Star Tomato Tuna Salad • Whole-grain bread	• Red Hot Fusilli • Tossed salad	• Rockport Fish Chowder • Sliced tomatoes • Whole-grain roll	• Zucchini Lasagne • Tossed salad	• Simple Greek Salad	• Cannery Row Soup • Tossed green salad	• Glorious Gazpacho • Staminator Shrimp Salad

Monday	Tuesday	Wednesday	Thursday	Friday	Saturday	Sunday
SNACK						
• Almonds and raisins	• Nut butter on rice cake	• Walnuts and raisins	• Almonds and figs	• Nut butter on celery sticks	• Dates and almonds	• Peanut butter and peach butter on Krisp bread
DINNER						
• Scrumptious Meat Loaf • Spicy Crunchy Salad • Compote Tropicale	• Black Bean and Onion Soup • Spinach-Sole Roll-Ups • Black Beans with Rice • Maple-Poached Pears	• Guiltless Quesadillas • Finger-Licking Curried Chicken • Rice with almonds • Sautéed kale • Rainbow Honey-Glazed Fruit Salad	• Zesty Beef with Broccoli • Smothered Greens • Baked sweet potatoes • Cupid's Quiver	• Baked trout amandine • Summer squash • Steamed carrots • Blackberry Cobbler • Four Play Fruit Medley	• Black skillet beef with greens and red potatoes • Whole-grain bread • Sliced tomatoes • Sliced mango	• Chicken Marsala • Green bean sauté • Tossed green salad
SNACK						
• Plain yogurt with berries	• Almonds and raisins	• Virgin Mary	• Pomegranate spritzer	• Crudités with yogurt dip	• Frozen banana	• Apple and sliced cheese

8

Eat, Drink, and Be Merry

Recipes for Great Food, Great Sex

To eat is a necessity, but to eat intelligently is an art.

—LA ROCHEFOUCAULD

The majority of our recipes are courtesy of the National Heart, Lung, and Blood Institute (NHLBI) Stay Young at Heart Program.* The Internet offers a wide range of recipes from gourmet to on-the-go. We encourage you to try any that are high in fruits and/or vegetables. When choosing protein, lean and mean is the way to go.

A GUIDE TO TYPICAL SERVING SIZES

For starches (grains, beans, and starchy vegetables), a serving can equal:

- 1 slice of bread.
- 1 small potato.

*Source: The National Heart, Lung, and Blood Institute, a part of the National Institute of Health and the US Department of Health and Human Services.

- ½ cup cooked cereal or ¾ cup dry cereal.

- ⅓ cup rice.

- ½ cup peas.

   For fruits, a typical serving might equal:

- 1 small apple.

- ½ cup apple or orange juice.

- ½ grapefruit.

- ½ banana.

- 1¼ cup whole strawberries.

·   For vegetables, a serving can equal:

- ½ cup carrots.

- ½ cup cooked green beans.

- 1 cup salad.

- ½ cup broccoli.

- ½ cup tomato juice.

A single serving of milk or yogurt equals 1 cup of fat-free plain yogurt or 1 cup of skim milk.

A single serving of protein foods, such as meat or cheese, is generally 2 to 3 ounces after cooking (this is about the size of a deck of cards).

Two ounces of cheese or 4 ounces of tofu (about ½ cup) equals a single serving of protein.

A single serving of oil is 1 teaspoon; a single serving of salad dressing is 1 tablespoon.

TABLE 8.1
Common Cooking Equivalents

1/16 cup (c) =	1 tablespoon
1/8 cup =	2 tablespoons
1/6 cup =	2 tablespoons + 2 teaspoons
1/4 cup =	4 tablespoons
1/3 cup =	5 tablespoons + 1 teaspoon
3/8 cup =	6 tablespoons
1/2 cup =	8 tablespoons
2/3 cup =	10 tablespoons + 2 teaspoons
3/4 cup =	12 tablespoons
1 cup =	48 teaspoons
1 cup =	16 tablespoons
8 fluid ounces (fl oz) =	1 cup
1 pint (pt) =	2 cups
1 quart (qt) =	2 pints
4 cups =	1 quart
1 gallon (gal) =	4 quarts
16 ounces (oz) =	1 pound (lb)
1 milliliter (ml) =	1 cubic centimeter (cc)
1 inch (in) =	2.54 centimeters (cm)

TABLE 8.2

Metric Conversion Factors

Multiply	By	To Get
Fluid ounces	29.57	grams
Ounces (dry)	28.35	grams
Grams	0.0353	ounces
Grams	0.0022	pounds
Kilograms	2.21	pounds
Pounds	453.6	grams
Pounds	0.4536	kilograms
Quarts	0.946	liters
Quarts (dry)	67.2	cubic inches
Quarts (liquid)	57.7	cubic inches
Liters	1.0567	quarts
Gallons	3,785	cubic centimeters
Gallons	3.785	liters

Frisky Veggie Frittata

MAKES 4 SERVINGS

Olive oil cooking spray
½ medium red onion, coarsely chopped
3 medium cloves garlic, finely chopped or pressed
2 cups zucchini, sliced into strips
2 ounces canned diced green jalapeño chilies
1 small tomato, chopped with excess pulp removed
2 Tbsp chopped fresh cilantro
2 whole eggs
4 egg whites
2 Tbsp chopped fresh parsley

Spray 8-10 inch omelet pan with olive oil, and heat. Add onion and garlic and sauté till onion is translucent.

Add remaining vegetables and cilantro, stir frequently, and sauté until zucchini is soft.

Beat whole eggs till frothy. In a separate glass bowl, beat egg whites till peaks form. Gently fold eggwhites into egg yolks.

Pour egg mixture into pan, covering the vegetable mixture. Reduce heat to low and cover the omelet. Cook until firm (about 10 minutes), being careful to lift edges of omelet with a spatual and tilt pan so any uncooked eggs run beneath vegetables.

When fully cooked, carefully run a spatula around edges and slide frittata onto a warm serving dish. Cut into quarters, garnish with parsley and serve.

Calories: 85	Sodium: 250 mg
Total fat: 2.7 g	Calcium: 34 mg
Saturated fat: .81 g	Iron: .86 mg
Cholesterol: 31 mg	

Good Morning Muesli

MAKES 4 SERVINGS

2 cups sliced raw almonds
2 cups oats, quick or old-fashioned
4 tsp raisins
4 cups low-fat plain yogurt
1 tsp pure vanilla extract
1 cup raw apple slices
1 cup sliced fresh strawberries

Preheat oven to 325° F. Place almonds on baking sheet and toast for 5 to 10 minutes. Remove almonds and spread oatmeal on baking sheet. Toast oatmeal for 5 to 10 minutes. Mix oatmeal, almonds, and raisins together, cool, and store in airtight container.

1 hour before serving, mix yogurt with vanilla and add dry mixture of oats, raisins, and almonds. Let sit in refrigerator. Garnish with fresh fruit and serve.

Calories: 614	Sodium: 176 mg
Total fat: 18.3 g	Fiber: 12.5 g
Saturated fat: 4.2 g	Cholesterol: 15 mg

Banana Berry Smoothie

4 ice cubes
1 cup crushed pineapple, canned in unsweetened juice
1 tsp vanilla extract
6 medium strawberries
1 medium banana, sliced
1 cup plain nonfat yogurt

Place ice cubes in blender and blend till crushed. Add pineapple, vanilla extract, 5 strawberries, banana, and yogurt. Blend well. Pour into tall glasses and garnish with strawberry slices.

Calories: 121

Fat: Less than 1 g

Saturated fat: Less than 1 g

Sodium: 64 mg

Cholesterol: 1 mg

Breakfast Burrito

Olive oil cooking spray
1 flour tortilla
½ cup egg substitute
1 Tbsp cooked kidney beans
1 ounce grated Cheddar or Monterey Jack cheese
1 Tbsp chunky salsa

Warm cast-iron frying pan. Spray with olive oil and place tortilla in pan. Brown for 2 to 3 minutes, turn over, and brown other side. Remove from pan.

Whisk egg substitute and scramble in pan. Spoon egg onto tortilla, top with beans, cheese, and salsa. Roll up and serve.

Calories: 323	Cholesterol: 32 mg
Fat: 15.6 g	Saturated fat: 7.3 g
Protein: 25.6 g	Sodium: 668 mg

Mango For It

2 ice cubes
4 Tbsp frozen mango juice (or 1 fresh pitted mango)
1 small banana, sliced
2 cups low-fat milk

Put ice cubes in blender and blend till crushed. Add mango juice or fruits. Blend 1 minute. Add milk and blend till fully mixed. Serve immediately.

VARIATIONS: May be made with orange juice, fresh papaya, or fresh strawberries.

Calories: 106

Total fat: 2 g

Saturated fat: 1 g

Cholesterol: 5 mg

Sodium: 63 mg

Calcium: 157 mg

Iron: Less than 1 mg

Curtido Cabbage Salvadore

MAKES 8 SERVINGS—SERVING SIZE: 1 CUP

1 medium head cabbage, chopped
2 small carrots, grated
1 small onion, sliced
½ tsp dried red pepper (optional)
½ tsp oregano
1 tsp olive oil
1 tsp salt
1 tsp brown sugar
¼ cup vinegar
½ cup water

Blanch cabbage in boiling water for 1 minute. Discard water.

Place cabbage in large bowl and add grated carrots, sliced onion, red pepper, oregano, olive oil, salt, brown sugar, vinegar, and water.

Place in refrigerator for at least 2 hours before serving.

---

*Calories: 41
Total fat: 1 g
Saturated fat: Less than 1 g
Cholesterol: 0 mg

Sodium: 293 mg
Calcium: 44 mg
Iron: 1 mg

Star Tomato Tuna Salad

2 6-ounce cans water-packed tuna
½ cup chopped raw celery
⅓ cup chopped green onions
6½ Tbsp reduced-fat mayonnaise
Dash of Worcestershire sauce
5 tomatoes

Tuna salad

Drain tuna. Flake with fork. Add celery, onion, mayonnaise and worcestershire sauce and mix well.

Tomato stars

Core tomatoes, taking care not to cut through to bottom. Slice as if making quarters, but leave sections attached. Gently spread apart and spoon tuna salad into opening.

Calories: 562
Total fat: 7 g
Saturated fat: 0 g

Cholesterol: 25 mg
Sodium: 238 mg

Tropical Shrimp Salad

1 clove garlic
3 Tbsp fresh lemon juice
⅛ tsp chili powder
1 tsp Worcestershire sauce
1 pound raw shrimp, peeled
1 medium head red cabbage, grated
1 carrot, grated
1 cup chopped watercress
⅓ cup lime juice
2 Tbsp honey
2 Tbsp chopped fresh basil
2 Tbsp chopped roasted peanuts
2 ripe red tomatoes, quartered

Combine garlic clove, lemon juice, chili powder, and Worcestershire sauce in blender and blend until smooth. Add shrimp and marinate for 1 hour.

Toss cabbage, carrots, and watercress together in bowl. Whisk together lime juice and honey and toss with vegetables.

Spray medium frying pan with olive oil and sauté shrimp in marinade until shrimp become firm and pink (approximately 3 minutes). Remove from pan and cool.

Place vegetable salad on large platter. Layer with shrimp and top with basil and peanuts. Garnish edges of platter with cut tomatoes.

Calories: 265	Fiber: 2 g
Protein: 26 g	Sodium: 188 mg
Fat: 4 g	

Fresh Cabbage and Tomato Salad

1 small head cabbage, sliced thinly
2 medium tomatoes, cut in cubes
1 cup sliced radishes
¼ tsp salt
2 tsp olive oil
2 Tbsp rice vinegar (or lemon juice)
½ tsp black pepper
½ tsp red pepper
2 Tbsp chopped fresh cilantro

In large bowl, mix together cabbage, tomatoes, and radishes.

In another bowl, mix together rest of ingredients and pour over vegetables.

---

*Calories: 41	Sodium: 88 mg
Total fat: 1 g	Calcium: 49 mg
Saturated fat: Less than 1 g	Iron: 1 mg
Cholesterol: 0 mg	

Simple Greek Salad

Salad
- 1 green bell pepper
- 1 red bell pepper
- 2 large tomatoes
- 1 cucumber
- 1 red onion
- 1 head romaine lettuce, well rinsed
- 6 ounces assorted olives (black and green)
- 1 cup crumbled feta cheese

Dressing
- 2 cloves garlic
- 6 Tbsp olive oil
- Juice of 1 lemon
- 1 tsp dried oregano
- Ground black pepper to taste

Coarsely chop green and red peppers, tomatoes, and cucumber. Cut onion in half. Chop half into small pieces and mix with peppers, tomatoes, and cucumber.

Line salad bowl with 3–4 large leaves of romaine lettuce. Tear remaining leaves into large pieces and toss with chopped vegetables. Place on top of lettuce leaves.

Thinly slice remaining onion and layer on chopped vegetables. Sprinkle olives and feta cheese on top of vegetable mixure.

Mince garlic or press through garlic press. Whisk together olive oil and lemon juice until cloudy. Add garlic, oregano, and black pepper and mix well. Drizzle over salad and serve.

Calories: 265   Sodium: 539 mg

Total fat: 22.4 g   Carbohydrates: 14 g

Saturated fat: 6 g   Protein: 6.3 g

Staminator Shrimp Salad

MAKES 6 SERVINGS

2 pounds shrimp, steamed
1 bunch fresh parsley
1 bunch green onions
2 cloves garlic
1 can black beans, drained and rinsed
3 Tbsp olive oil
Juice of large lemon
1 cup grated Parmesan cheese
Salad greens
1 cup cherry tomatoes

Chop shrimp into large pieces. Chop parsley, green onions, and garlic and toss together with shrimp and beans. Whisk olive oil, lemon juice, and Parmesan cheese together, pour over shrimp mixture, and lightly toss. Place salad greens in large salad bowl, place shrimp mixture on top, and garnish with cherry tomatoes.

Calories: 183   Fiber: 3.6 g

Carbohydrates: 11 g   Protein: 12 g

Cholesterol: 45 mg   Sodium: 270 mg

Total Fat: 10 g   Saturated fat: 3 g

Spicy Crunchy Salad

MAKES 1 SERVING

¾ cup small broccoli florets
¾ cup small cauliflower florets
½ cup carrot, sliced in rounds
⅛ tsp salt
¼ tsp ground ginger
¼ tsp ground cumin
⅛ tsp ground coriander
⅛ tsp ground nutmeg
⅛ tsp chili powder
½ tsp honey
3 Tbsp fat-free sour cream
2 tsp cider vinegar
2 Tbsp scallions

Place broccoli, cauliflower, and carrots in steamer over 1 cup boiling water. Steam for 5 minutes.

Place spices in small cast-iron frying pan; cook over medium heat until lightly browned, stirring constantly.

Chop scallions and set aside. Combine sour cream, vinegar, and honey in bowl and whisk till thoroughly blended. Add spices and whisk again. Add steamed vegetables and stir until all pieces are thoroughly coated. Sprinkle with chopped scallions.

Calories: 57	Carbohydrates: 10.7 g
Total fat: 0.4 g	Fiber: 3 g
Cholesterol: 0 mg	Sodium: 194 mg
Protein: 3.8 g	Calcium: 40 mg

Sassy Salsa

3 large tomatoes
1 medium onion,
2 serrano or jalapeño peppers
1 clove garlic
3 Tbsp chopped cilantro
⅛ tsp dried oregano
⅛ tsp salt
⅛ tsp pepper
½ ripe avocado
Juice of 1 lime

Chop tomatoes and onion into small pieces. Chop peppers and garlic into fine pieces. Mix together with cilantro, oregano, salt, and pepper. Chop avocado, mix with lime juice, and toss with tomato mixture. Serve immediately. Can be refrigerated up to 4–5 hours.

Calories: 42

Total fat: 2 g

Saturated fat: Less than 1 g

Cholesterol: 0 mg

Sodium: 44 mg

Calcium: 12 mg

Iron: 1 mg

Easy Vinaigrette Salad Dressing

2 cloves fresh garlic
1 Tbsp red wine vinegar
¼ tsp honey
1 Tbsp virgin olive oil
¼ tsp black pepper

Put garlic through garlic press or chop finely. Pour vinegar, honey, and oil into glass jar with lid. Shake till thoroughly mixed. Add garlic and pepper. Shake just before using.

Calories: 33

Total fat: 3 g

Saturated fat: Less than 1 g

Cholesterol: 0 mg

Sodium: 0 mg

Creamy Yogurt Dressing

8 ounces plain nonfat yogurt
¼ cup nonfat mayonnaise
2 Tbsp dried chives
2 Tbsp dried dill
2 Tbsp lemon juice

Whisk yogurt and mayonnaise together till well blended. Stir in herbs and lemon juice. Serve immediately or refrigerate.

Calories: 23

Total fat: 0 g

Saturated fat: Less than 0 g

Cholesterol: 1 mg

Sodium: 84 mg

Glorious Gazpacho

MAKES 6 SERVINGS—SERVING SIZE: 1 CUP

4 cups tomato juice (low-sodium, if desired)
1 clove garlic, minced
hot pepper sauce to taste
2 Tbsp olive oil
⅛ tsp cayenne pepper
½ tsp Worcestershire sauce
¼ tsp black pepper
½ medium onion, peeled and coarsely chopped
1 small green pepper, peeled, cored, seeded, and coarsely chopped
1 small cucumber, peeled, pared, seeded, and coarsely chopped
1 large tomato, finely diced
1 lemon, thinly sliced
2 Tbsp minced chives or scallion tops

Put tomato juice, garlic, hot sauce, olive oil, cayenne, Worcestershire sauce, and black pepper in blender for 30 seconds. Add chopped onion, pepper, cucumber, and tomato. Buzz blender off and on 3–4 times to mix through.

Chill thoroughly. Garnish with lemon slices and chives.

Calories: 87

Total fat: 5 g

Saturated fat: less than 1 g

Cholesterol: 0 mg

Sodium: 593 mg (less with low-sodium tomato juice)

Cannery Row Soup

2 Tbsp olive oil
1 clove garlic, minced
3 carrots, cut in thin strips
2 cup celery, sliced
½ cup onion, chopped
¼ cup green pepper, chopped
1 can (28-ounce) whole tomatoes, cut up, with liquid
1 cup clam juice
¼ tsp dried thyme, crushed
¼ tsp dried basil, crushed
⅛ tsp black pepper
2 pounds varied fish fillets (haddock, perch, flounder, cod, sole, etc.),
    cut into 1-inch-square cubes
¼ cup fresh parsley, minced

Heat oil in large sauce pan. Sauté garlic, carrots, celery, onion, and green pepper in oil 3 minutes.

Add remaining ingredients except parsley and fish. Cover and simmer 10 to 15 minutes or until vegetables are fork tender.

Add fish and parsley. Simmer, covered, 5 to 10 minutes more or until fish flakes easily and is opaque. Serve hot.

---

*Calories: 170
Total Fat: 5 g
Saturated fat: Less than 1 g

Cholesterol: 56 mg
Sodium: 380 mg

Meatball Soup

10 cups water
1 Tbsp annato (achiote)
1 bay leaf
1 small onion, chopped
½ cup chopped green pepper
1 tsp mint (yerbabuena)
½ pound ground chicken
½ pound ground lean beef
2 small tomatoes, chopped
½ tsp oregano
4 Tbsp instant corn flour (masa harina)
½ tsp black pepper
2 cloves garlic, minced
½ tsp salt
2 medium carrots, chopped
1 medium chayote (christophine), chopped
2 cups cabbage, chopped
2 celery stalks, chopped
1 (10-ounce) package frozen corn
2 medium zucchini, chopped
½ cup minced cilantro

In large pot, combine water, annato, bay leaf, half the onion, all of the green pepper, and mint. Bring to a boil.

In bowl, combine chicken and beef, the other half of the onion, tomato, oregano, corn flour, pepper, garlic, and salt. Mix well. Form 1-inch meatballs. Place meatballs in boiling water and lower heat. Cook over low heat for 30 to 45 minutes.

Add carrots, chayote, cabbage, and celery. Cook over low heat for 25 minutes. Add corn and zucchini and cook for another 5 minutes. Garnish with cilantro and the rest of the mint.

---

*Calories: 161

Total fat: 4 g

Saturated fat: 1 g

Cholesterol: 31 mg

Sodium: 193 mg

Calcium: 47 mg

Iron: 2 mg

Bean and Macaroni Soup

2 (16-ounce) cans great northern beans
1 Tbsp olive oil
½ pound fresh mushrooms, sliced
1 cup coarsely chopped onion
2 cups sliced carrots
1 cup coarsely chopped celery
1 clove garlic, minced
3 cups cut-up peeled fresh tomatoes or 1½ pounds canned whole
    tomatoes, cut up
1 tsp dried sage
1 tsp dried thyme
½ tsp dried oregano
Black pepper to taste
1 bay leaf, crumbled
1 pound uncooked elbow macaroni

Drain beans and reserve liquid. Rinse beans.

Heat oil in 6-quart kettle; add mushrooms, onion, carrots, celery, and garlic, and sauté 5 minutes.

Add tomatoes, sage, thyme, oregano, pepper, and bay leaf. Cover and cook over medium heat 20 minutes.

Cook macaroni according to directions on package using unsalted water. Drain when cooked. Do not overcook.

Combine reserved bean liquid with water to make 4 cups.

Add liquid, beans, and cooked macaroni to vegetable mixture. Bring to boil; cover and simmer until soup is thoroughly heated, stirring occasionally.

*Calories: 158

Total fat: 1 g

Saturated fat: Less than 1 g

Cholesterol: 0 mg

Sodium: 154 mg (using canned
tomatoes, sodium would be higher)

Rockport Fish Chowder

2 Tbsp vegetable oil
¾ cup coarsely chopped onion
½ cup coarsely chopped celery
1 cup sliced carrots
2 cups raw, peeled and cubed potatoes
¼ tsp thyme
½ tsp paprika
2 cups bottled clam juice
8 whole peppercorns
1 bay leaf
1 pound fresh or frozen (thawed) cod or haddock fillets
¼ cup flour
3 cups 1% milk
1 Tbsp chopped fresh parsley

Heat oil in large saucepan. Add onion and celery and sauté about 3 minutes.

Add carrots, potatoes, thyme, paprika, and clam juice. Wrap peppercorns and bay leaf in cheesecloth. Add to pot. Bring to boil, reduce heat, and simmer 15 minutes.

Add fish and simmer an additional 15 minutes, or until fish flakes easily and is opaque.

Remove fish and vegetables; break fish into chunks. Bring broth to boil and continue boiling until volume is reduced to 1 cup. Remove bay leaf and peppercorns.

Shake flour and ½ cup milk in container with a tight-fitting lid until smooth. Add to broth in saucepan with remaining milk. Cook over medium heat, stirring constantly, until mixture boils and is thickened.

Return vegetables and fish chunks to stock and heat thoroughly. Serve hot, sprinkled with chopped parsley.

---

*Calories: 186

Total fat: 6 g

Saturated fat: 1 g

Cholesterol: 34 mg

Sodium: 302 mg

Guiltless Quesadillas

MAKES 8 SERVINGS—SERVING SIZE: ½ TORTILLA

1 red bell pepper
1 medium yellow squash
½ small onion
1 medium tomato
1 (16-ounce) can corn
2 tsp lime juice
¼ tsp chili powder
⅛ tsp pepper
1 cup shredded low-fat Monterey Jack cheese
4 6-inch corn tortillas
Olive oil spray
½ cup low-sodium salsa
½ cup nonfat or low-fat sour cream

Chop pepper, squash, and onion into small pieces. Spray cast-iron skillet with olive oil and sauté until onion is translucent and pepper is soft. Chop tomato into small pieces. Add corn and tomato to vegetable mixture and heat through. Remove from heat. Place vegetables in bowl.

Add lime juice and chili powder and stir through until vegetables are coated. Add shredded cheese and stir through.

Reheat pan for tortillas. Spray one side of tortilla with olive oil, place in pan, and lightly toast for 1 to 2 minutes. Place large spoonful of vegetable/cheese mixture on ½ of tortilla and fold tortilla over the filling. Cook for approximately 1 to 2 minutes, turn, and cook on other side until tortilla is gently browned and cheese has melted inside. Place on cutting board and repeat process with remaining tortillas.

To serve, cut quesadillas in half and place on a serving platter. Top each quesadilla with 1 tablespoon each of salsa and sour cream.

Calories: 183

Cholesterol: 9 mg

Fat: 4 g

Saturated fat: 2 g

Sodium: 161 mg

Virgin Mary

MAKES 1 SERVING

4 ounces tomato juice

2–3 dashes lemon juice

1 pinch celery salt

4–6 drops Worcestershire sauce

1 pinch coarse pepper

2–3 drops Tabasco sauce

1 celery stalk

Pour tomato juice over ice cubes in large highball glass. Season to taste with lemon, celery salt, Worcestershire, pepper, and Tabasco. Stir and garnish with celery. Serve in highball glass.

Calories: 22

Carbohydrates: 5.8 g

Sodium: 35 mg

Cholesterol: 0 mg

Scrumptious Meat Loaf

MAKES 6 SERVINGS—SERVING SIZE: 1 ¼-INCH-THICK SLICE

1 pound extra-lean ground beef or turkey
½ cup (4 ounces) tomato paste
¼ cup chopped onion
¼ cup chopped green pepper
¼ cup chopped red pepper
1 cup fresh, blanched, chopped tomatoes
½ tsp low-sodium mustard
¼ tsp ground black pepper
½ tsp chopped hot pepper
2 cloves garlic, chopped
2 stalks scallion, chopped
½ tsp ground ginger
⅛ tsp ground nutmeg
1 tsp grated orange rind
½ tsp crushed thyme
¼ cup finely grated bread crumbs

Mix all ingredients together.

Place in 1-pound loaf pan (preferably with drip rack) and bake covered at 350° F for 50 minutes. Uncover pan and continue baking for 12 minutes.

---

*Calories: 193

Fat: 9 g

Saturated fat: 3 g

Cholesterol: 45 mg

Sodium: 91 mg

Zesty Beef with Broccoli

¼ cup all-purpose flour
1 10-ounce can beef broth
2 Tbsp soy sauce
2 Tbsp honey
1 clove garlic, minced
¼ tsp chopped fresh gingerroot
1 pound boneless round steak, cut into bite-sized pieces
4 cups chopped fresh broccoli

In small saucepan, heat broth with flour soy sauce and honey. Add garlic and ginger and cook 2 minutes until garlic is soft.

In large skillet or wok over high heat, cook steak pieces until browned, stirring frequently. Stir in broth mixture. Add broccoli and bring to boil. Reduce heat and cook 5 to 10 minutes.

Calories: 189
Protein: 15 g
Fat: 7 g

Carbohydrate: 18 g
Cholesterol: 31 mg

Chicken Orientale

8 boneless, skinless chicken breasts, quartered
Black pepper to taste
8 fresh mushrooms
8 parboiled whole white onions
2 oranges, quartered
8 canned pineapple chunks
8 cherry tomatoes
1 (6-ounce) can frozen concentrated apple juice, thawed
1 cup dry white wine
2 Tbsp low-sodium soy sauce
Dash ground ginger
2 Tbsp vinegar
¼ cup vegetable oil

Sprinkle chicken breasts with pepper.

Thread 8 skewers as follows: chicken, mushroom, chicken, onion, chicken, orange quarter, chicken, pineapple chunk, chicken, cherry tomato.

Place kebabs in shallow pan.

Combine remaining ingredients; spoon over kebabs. Marinate in refrigerator at least 1 hour.

Preheat broiler.

Drain kebabs. Broil 6 inches from heat, 15 minutes on each side, brushing with marinade every 5 minutes. Discard any leftover marinade.

---

*Calories: 359	Cholesterol: 66 mg
Total fat: 11 g	Sodium: 226 mg
Saturated fat: 2 g	

Chicken Ratatouille

1 Tbsp vegetable oil

4 medium chicken breast halves, skinned, fat removed, boned, and cut into 1-inch pieces

2 zucchini, about 7 inches long, unpeeled and thinly sliced

1 small eggplant, peeled and cut into 1-inch cubes

1 medium onion, thinly sliced

1 medium green pepper, cut into 1-inch pieces

½ pound fresh mushrooms, sliced

1 (16-ounce) can whole tomatoes, cut up

1 clove garlic, minced

1½ tsp dried basil, crushed

1 Tbsp minced fresh parsley

Black pepper to taste

Heat oil in large nonstick skillet. Add chicken and sauté about 3 minutes, or until lightly browned.

Add zucchini, eggplant, onion, green pepper, and mushrooms. Cook about 15 minutes, stirring occasionally.

Add tomatoes, garlic, basil, parsley, and pepper; stir and continue cooking about 5 minutes, or until chicken is tender.

Preheat broiler.

Broil 6 inches from heat, 15 minutes on each side, brushing with marinade every 5 minutes. Discard any leftover marinade.

---

*Calories: 266

Total fat: 8 g

Saturated fat: 2 g

Cholesterol: 66 mg

Sodium: 253 mg

Finger-Licking Curried Chicken

MAKES 6 SERVINGS—

SERVING SIZE: ½ BREAST OR 2 SMALL DRUMSTICKS

1½ tsp curry powder
1 tsp crushed thyme
1 stalk scallion, chopped
1 Tbsp chopped hot pepper
¼ tsp cayenne pepper
1 tsp ground black pepper
8 cloves garlic, crushed
1 Tbsp grated ginger
¾ tsp salt
8 pieces chicken, skinless (breast, drumstick)
1 Tbsp olive oil
1 cup water
1 medium white potato, diced
1 large onion, chopped

Mix together curry powder, thyme, scallion, hot pepper, cayenne pepper, black pepper, garlic, ginger, and salt.

Sprinkle seasoning mixture on chicken. Marinate at least 2 hours in the refrigerator.

Heat oil in skillet over medium flame. Add chicken and sauté. Add water and allow chicken to cook over medium flame 30 minutes. Add diced potato and cook an additional 30 minutes. Add onion and cook 15 minutes more or until meat is tender.

---

*Calories: 213	Cholesterol: 81 mg
Fat: 6 g	Sodium: 363 mg

Very Lemony Chicken

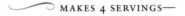
1½ pounds chicken breast, skinned and fat removed
½ cup fresh lemon juice
2 Tbsp white wine vinegar
½ cup fresh sliced lemon peel
3 tsp chopped fresh oregano or 1 tsp dried oregano,
    crushed
1 medium onion, sliced
¼ tsp salt
Black pepper to taste
½ tsp paprika

Place chicken in 13x9x2-inch glass baking dish.

Mix lemon juice, vinegar, lemon peel, oregano, and onion. Pour over chicken, cover, and marinate in refrigerator several hours or overnight, turning occasionally.

Preheat oven to 325° F.

Sprinkle chicken with salt, pepper, and paprika.

Cover and bake 30 minutes. Uncover and bake 30 minutes more or until done.

---

*Calories: 154
Total fat: 5 g
Saturated fat: 2 g

Cholesterol: 63 mg
Sodium: 202 mg

Chicken Marsala

⅛ tsp black pepper

¼ tsp salt

¼ cup flour

4 chicken breasts (5 ounces each), boned, skinless

1 Tbsp olive oil

½ cup Marsala wine

½ cup chicken stock, fat skimmed from top

½ lemon of fresh lemon juice

½ cup sliced mushrooms

1 Tbsp chopped fresh parsley

Mix together pepper, salt, and flour. Coat chicken with seasoned flour.

In heavy-bottomed skillet, heat oil. Place chicken breasts in skillet and brown on both sides. Remove chicken from skillet and set aside.

Add wine to skillet, and stir until wine is heated. Add stock, juice, and mushrooms. Stir to toss, reduce heat, and cook about 10 minutes until sauce is partially reduced.

Return browned chicken breasts to skillet. Spoon sauce over chicken. Cover and cook about 5 to 10 minutes or until chicken is done.

Serve sauce over chicken. Garnish with chopped parsley.

---

*Calories: 277
Total fat: 8 g
Saturated fat: 2 g

Cholesterol: 77 mg
Sodium: 304 mg

Scallop Kebabs

3 medium green peppers, cut into 1½-inch squares
1½ pounds fresh bay scallops
1 pint cherry tomatoes
¼ cup dry white wine
¼ cup vegetable oil
3 Tbsp lemon juice
Dash garlic powder
Black pepper to taste

Parboil green peppers for 2 minutes.

Alternately thread first 3 ingredients on skewers.

Combine next 5 ingredients. Brush kebabs with wine-oil-lemon mixture.

Place on grill (or under broiler). Grill 15 minutes, turning and basting frequently.

---

*Calories: 224

Total fat: 6 g

Saturated fat: Less than 1 g

Cholesterol: 43 mg

Sodium: 355 mg

Mediterranean Baked Fish

2 tsp olive oil
1 large onion, sliced
1 (16-ounce) can whole tomatoes, drained (reserve juice)
  and coarsely chopped
1 bay leaf
1 clove garlic, minced
1 cup dry white wine
½ cup reserved tomato juice, from canned tomatoes
¼ cup lemon juice
¼ cup orange juice
1 Tbsp fresh grated orange peel
1 tsp fennel seeds, crushed
½ tsp dried oregano, crushed
½ tsp dried thyme, crushed
½ tsp dried basil, crushed
Black pepper to taste
1 pound fish fillets (sole, flounder, or sea perch)

Heat oil in large nonstick skillet. Add onion, and sauté over moderate heat 5 minutes or until soft.

Add all remaining ingredients except fish. Stir well and simmer 30 minutes, uncovered.

Preheat oven to 375° F.

Arrange fish in 10x6-inch baking dish; cover with sauce.

Bake, uncovered, about 15 minutes or until fish flakes easily and is opaque.

*Calories: 177

Cholesterol: 56 mg

Total fat: 4 g

Sodium: 281 mg

Saturated fat: 1 g

Baked Trout Olé

MAKES 6 SERVINGS—SERVING SIZE: 1 PIECE

2 pounds trout fillet, cut into 6 pieces (any kind of fish can be used)
3 Tbsp lime juice (about 2 limes)
1 medium tomato, chopped
½ medium onion, chopped
3 Tbsp chopped cilantro
½ tsp olive oil
¼ tsp black pepper
¼ tsp salt
¼ tsp red pepper (optional)

Preheat oven to 350° F.

Rinse fish and pat dry. Place in baking dish.

In separate dish, mix remaining ingredients together and pour over fish.

Bake 15 to 20 minutes or until fork-tender.

*Calories: 230

Sodium: 162 mg

Total fat: 9 g

Calcium: 60 mg

Saturated fat: 2 g

Iron: 1 mg

Cholesterol: 58 mg

Spinach Sole Roll-Ups

Nonstick cooking spray (as needed)
1 tsp olive oil
½ pound fresh mushrooms, sliced
½ pound fresh spinach, chopped
1 clove garlic, minced
¼ tsp crushed oregano leaves
1½ pounds sole fillets or other white fish
2 Tbsp sherry
4 ounces (1 cup) part-skim mozzarella cheese, grated
Wooden toothpicks

Preheat oven to 400° F. Spray 10x6-inch baking dish with olive oil.

Add olive oil to skillet and heat. Add mushrooms and stir till coated with oil. Cover pan and cook gently about 3 minutes. Add spinach, stir through, and cook uncovered about 1 minute. Add garlic and oregano to mixture and stir through.

Remove vegetable mixture from heat, and drain any liquid into baking dish. Place fish fillets on cutting board.

Divide vegetable mixture evenly among fillets, spreading mixture over length of fillet. Roll up each fillet, secure with wooden toothpick, and place in baking dish. Roll fillet around mixture and place seam-side down in prepared baking dish. Sprinkle fillets with sherry and top with grated cheese. Place dish in oven and bake 15 to 20 minutes.

Calories: 262	Cholesterol: 95 mg
Total fat: 8 g	Sodium: 312 mg
Saturated fat: 4 g	

Black Beans with Rice

MAKES 6 SERVINGS—SERVING SIZE: 8 OUNCES

1 pound dry black beans
7 cups water
1 medium green pepper, coarsely chopped
1½ cups chopped onion
1 Tbsp vegetable oil
2 bay leaves
1 clove garlic, minced
½ tsp salt
1 Tbsp vinegar or lemon juice
6 cups rice, cooked in unsalted water
1 (4-ounce) jar sliced pimiento, drained
1 lemon, cut into wedges

Pick through beans to remove bad beans. Soak overnight in cold water. Drain and rinse.

In large soup pot or Dutch oven, stir together beans, water, green pepper, onion, oil, bay leaves, garlic, and salt. Cover and boil 1 hour.

Reduce heat and simmer, covered, 3 to 4 hours or until beans are very tender. Stir occasionally and add water if needed.

Remove about ⅓ of the beans, mash, and return to pot. Stir and heat through. Remove bay leaves and stir in vinegar or lemon juice when ready to serve.

Serve over rice. Garnish with sliced pimiento and lemon wedges.

---

*Calories: 561

Total fat: 4 g

Saturated fat: 1 g

Cholesterol: 0 mg

Sodium: 193 mg

New Orleans Red Beans

MAKES 8 SERVINGS—SERVING SIZE: 1¼ CUPS

1 pound dry red beans
2 quarts water
1½ cups chopped onion
1 cup chopped celery
4 bay leaves
1 cup chopped green pepper
3 Tbsp chopped garlic
3 Tbsp chopped parsley
2 tsp dried thyme, crushed
1 tsp salt
1 tsp black pepper

Pick through beans to remove bad beans; rinse thoroughly.

In large pot, combine beans, water, onion, celery, and bay leaves. Bring to boil; reduce heat. Cover and cook over low heat for about 1½ hours or until beans are tender. Stir. Mash beans against side of pan.

Add green pepper, garlic, parsley, thyme, salt, and black pepper. Cook, uncovered, over low heat until creamy, about 30 minutes. Remove bay leaves. Serve with hot cooked brown rice, if desired.

*Calories: 171	Cholesterol: 0 mg
Total fat: Less than 1 g	Sodium: 285 mg
Saturated fat: Less than 1 g	

Summer Vegetable Spaghetti

MAKES 9 SERVINGS—SERVING SIZE: 1 CUP SPAGHETTI AND ¾ CUP SAUCE WITH VEGETABLES

2 cups small yellow onions, cut into eighths

2 cups (about 1 pound) chopped, peeled, fresh, ripe tomatoes

2 cups (about 1 pound) thinly sliced yellow and green squash

1½ cups (about ½ pound) cut fresh green beans

⅔ cup water

2 Tbsp minced fresh parsley

1 clove garlic, minced

½ tsp chili powder

¼ tsp salt

Black pepper to taste

1 (6-ounce) can tomato paste

1 pound uncooked spaghetti

½ cup grated Parmesan cheese

Combine first 10 ingredients in large saucepan; cook 10 minutes, then stir in tomato paste. Cover and cook gently, 15 minutes, stirring occasionally until vegetables are tender.

Cook spaghetti in unsalted water according to package directions.

Spoon sauce over drained hot spaghetti and sprinkle Parmesan cheese over top.

---

*Calories: 279

Total fat: 3 g

Saturated fat: 1 g

Cholesterol: 4 mg

Sodium: 173 mg

Zucchini Lasagne

¾ cup grated part-skim mozzarella cheese

¼ cup grated Parmesan cheese

1½ cups fat-free cottage cheese

2½ cups tomato sauce, no salt added

1½ cups sliced raw zucchini

2 tsp dried basil

2 tsp dried oregano

¼ cup chopped onion

1 clove garlic

⅛ tsp black pepper

½ pound lasagne noodles, cooked in unsalted water

Preheat oven to 350° F. Lightly spray 9x13-inch baking dish with vegetable oil spray.

In small bowl, combine ⅛ cup mozzarella and 1 Tbsp Parmesan cheese. Set aside.

In medium bowl, combine remaining mozzarella and Parmesan with all of the cottage cheese. Mix well and set aside.

Combine tomato sauce with remaining ingredients except zucchini and noodles. Spread thin layer of tomato sauce in bottom of baking dish. Add a third of the noodles in a single layer.

Spread half the cottage cheese mixture on top. Add a layer of zucchini. Repeat layering.

Add a thin coating of sauce. Top with noodles, sauce, and reserved cheese mixture. Cover with aluminum foil.

Bake 30 to 40 minutes. Cool 10 to 15 minutes. Cut into 6 portions.

*Calories: 276   Cholesterol: 11 mg

Total Fat: 5 g   Sodium: 380 mg

Saturated fat: 2 g

Italian Vegetable Bake

MAKES 8 SERVINGS—SERVING SIZE: ½ CUP

1 (28-ounce) can whole tomatoes

1 medium onion, sliced

½ pound fresh green beans, sliced

½ pound fresh okra, cut into ½-inch pieces, or half a 10-ounce
*   package (¾ cup)*

¾ cup finely chopped green pepper

2 Tbsp lemon juice

1 tsp chopped fresh basil, or 1 tsp dried basil, crushed

1½ tsp chopped fresh oregano leaves, or ½ tsp dried oregano, crushed

3 medium (7-inch-long) zucchini, cut into 1-inch cubes

1 medium eggplant, pared and cut into 1-inch cubes

2 Tbsp grated Parmesan cheese

Preheat oven to 325° F.

Drain and coarsely chop tomatoes. Save liquid. Mix together tomatoes and reserved liquid, onion, green beans, okra, green pepper, lemon juice, and herbs. Cover and bake 15 minutes.

Mix in zucchini and eggplant and continue baking, covered, 60 to 70 more minutes or until vegetables are tender. Stir occasionally.

Sprinkle top with Parmesan cheese just before serving.

*Calories: 36   Cholesterol: Less than 1 mg

Total fat: Less than 1 g   Sodium: 86 mg

Saturated fat: Less than 1 g

Smothered Greens

3 cups water
¼ pound smoked turkey breast, skinless, cut into bite-sized pieces
1 Tbsp freshly chopped hot pepper
¼ tsp cayenne pepper
¼ tsp ground cloves
2 cloves garlic, crushed
½ tsp thyme
1 stalk scallion, chopped
1 tsp ground ginger
¼ cup chopped onion
2 pounds greens (mustard, turnip, collard, kale, or mixture)

Place all ingredients except greens into large saucepan and bring to boil.

Prepare greens by washing thoroughly and removing stems. Tear or slice leaves into bite-sized pieces. Add greens to turkey stock. Cook 20 to 30 minutes until tender.

---

*Calories: 80

Fat 2: g

Saturated fat: Less than 1 g

Cholesterol: 16 mg

Sodium: 378 mg

Limas and Spinach

2 cups frozen lima beans
1 Tbsp vegetable oil
1 cup (4 ounces) fennel, cut in strips
½ cup chopped onion
¼ cup low-sodium chicken broth
4 cups leaf spinach, washed thoroughly
1 Tbsp distilled vinegar
⅛ tsp black pepper
1 Tbsp raw chives

Steam or boil lima beans in unsalted water approximately 10 minutes. Drain.

In skillet, sauté fennel and onion in oil. Add beans and broth, cover, and cook 2 minutes.

Stir in spinach. Cover and cook until spinach has wilted, about 2 minutes.

Stir in vinegar and pepper. Cover and let stand 30 seconds.

Sprinkle with chives and serve.

---

*Calories: 93

Fat: 2 g

Saturated fat: Less than 1 g

Cholesterol: 0 mg

Sodium: 84 mg

Red-Hot Fusilli

1 Tbsp olive oil
2 cloves garlic, minced
¼ cup freshly minced parsley, plus extra for garnish
4 cups chopped ripe tomatoes
1 Tbsp chopped fresh basil or 1 tsp dried basil
1 Tbsp crushed oregano leaves or 1 tsp dried oregano
¼ tsp salt
Ground red pepper or cayenne to taste
½ pound cooked chicken breasts, diced into ½-inch pieces
    (¾ pound raw) (optional)
8 ounces uncooked fusilli pasta (4 cups cooked)

Heat oil in medium saucepan. Sauté garlic and parsley until golden.

Add tomatoes and spices. Cook, uncovered, over low heat 15 minutes or until thickened, stirring frequently. If desired, add chicken and continue cooking 15 minutes until chicken is heated through and sauce is thick.

Cook pasta until firm in unsalted water.

To serve, spoon sauce over pasta and sprinkle with coarsely chopped parsley. Serve hot as a main dish and cold for the next day's lunch.

---

*Calories: 304   Cholesterol: 0 mg
Total fat: 5 g   Sodium: 285 mg
Saturated fat: Less than 1 g

With Chicken:
Calories: 398   Cholesterol: 44 mg
Total fat: 7 g   Sodium: 325 mg
Saturated fat: 1 g

Garlic Mashed Potatoes

1 pound (about 2 large) potatoes, peeled and quartered
2 cups skim milk
2 large cloves garlic, chopped
½ tsp white pepper

Stovetop Directions

Cook potatoes, covered, in small amount of boiling water for 20 to 25 minutes or until tender. Remove from heat. Drain and re-cover.

Meanwhile, in small saucepan over low heat, cook garlic in milk until soft, about 30 minutes.

Add milk-garlic mixture and white pepper to potatoes. Beat with electric mixer on low speed or mash with potato masher until smooth.

Microwave Directions

Scrub potatoes, pat dry, and prick with fork. On plate, cook potatoes, uncovered, on 100 percent power (high) until tender, about 12 minutes, turning potatoes over once. Let stand 5 minutes. Peel and quarter.

Meanwhile, in 4-cup glass measuring cup, combine milk and garlic. Cook, uncovered, on 50 percent power (medium) until garlic is soft, about 4 minutes. Continue as directed above.

---

*Calories: 141	Cholesterol: 2 mg
Total fat: Less than 1 g	Sodium: 70 mg
Saturated fat: Less than 1 g	

Oriental Rice

MAKES 10 SERVINGS—SERVING SIZE: ½ CUP

1½ cups water
1 cup chicken stock or broth, fat skimmed from top
1⅓ cups long-grain white rice, uncooked
2 tsp vegetable oil
2 Tbsp finely chopped onion
1 cup finely chopped celery
2 Tbsp finely chopped green pepper
½ cup chopped pecans
¼ tsp ground sage
½ cup sliced water chestnuts
¼ tsp nutmeg
Black pepper to taste

Bring water and stock to boil in medium saucepan. Add rice and stir. Cover and simmer 20 minutes. Remove pan from heat. Let stand, covered, 5 minutes or until all liquid is absorbed. Reserve.

Heat oil in large nonstick skillet. Sauté onion, celery, and green pepper over moderate heat 3 minutes. Stir in remaining ingredients, including reserved cooked rice. Fluff with fork before serving.

---

*Calories: 139

Total fat: 5 g

Saturated fat: Less than 1 g

Cholesterol: 0 mg

Sodium: 86 mg

Sunshine Rice

1½ Tbsp vegetable oil
1¼ cups finely chopped celery with leaves
½ cup finely chopped onion
1 cup water
½ cup orange juice
2 Tbsp lemon juice
Dash hot sauce
1 cup long-grain white rice, uncooked
¼ cup slivered almonds

Heat oil in medium saucepan. Add celery and onion and sauté until tender, about 10 minutes.

Add water, juices, and hot sauce. Bring to boil. Stir in rice and bring back to boil. Remove from heat and let stand, covered, until rice is tender and liquid is absorbed.

Stir in almonds. Serve immediately as side dish for fish entrée.

---

*Calories: 182	Cholesterol: 0 mg
Total fat: 7 g	Sodium: 21 mg
Saturated fat: Less than 1 g	

Rainbow Honey-Glazed Fruit Salad

MAKES 12 SERVINGS—SERVING SIZE: 4-OUNCE CUP

Fruit salad
  2 cups fresh blueberries
  2 cups seedless grapes
  2 cups fresh strawberries, halved
  2 bananas, sliced
  1 large mango, peeled and diced
  2 nectarines, unpeeled and sliced
  1 kiwi fruit, peeled and sliced

Honey Orange Sauce
  ⅓ cup unsweetened orange juice
  2 Tbsp lemon juice
  1½ Tbsp honey
  ¼ tsp ground ginger
  Dash nutmeg

Wash berries and grapes. Layer strawberries, bananas, blueberries, mango, and grapes in glass serving bowl. Layer slices of nectarines and kiwi on top. Combine orange juice, lemon juice, and honey in glass bowl and mix till honey is dissolved in juice. Add ginger and nutmeg. Drizzle sauce over fruit before serving.

Calories: 96

Total fat: 1 g

Saturated fat: Less than 1 g

Cholesterol: 0 mg

Sodium: 4 mg

Compote Tropicale

¾ cup water
½ cup honey
2 tsp fresh lemon juice
1 piece lemon peel
½ tsp rum or rum flavoring (optional)
1 pineapple, cored and peeled, cut into 8 slices
2 mangoes, peeled and pitted, cut into 8 pieces
3 bananas, peeled, cut into 8 diagonal pieces
Fresh mint leaves

In large saucepan, mix water with honey, lemon juice, and lemon peel (and rum extract if desired). Bring mixture to boil, reduce heat, and pour in fruit. Cook over very low heat for 5 minutes, stirring constantly. Drain off liquid and remove lemon peel.

Cool fruit mixture thoroughly. Place fruit in dessert glasses, pour syrup over fruit, and garnish with mint leaves.

Calories: 148	Sodium: 3 mg
Total fat: Less than 1 g	Calcium: 15 mg
Saturated fat: Less than 1 g	Iron: Less than 1 mg
Cholesterol: 0 mg	

Blackberry Cobbler

1 cup whole wheat flour
2 tsp. baking powder
1 cup brown sugar
¾ cup low-fat milk
½ tsp salt
2½ cups blackberries

Preheat oven to 400° F.

Mix flour, baking powder, ½ cup sugar, milk, and salt in glass bowl.

Lightly grease 9x16x2-inch baking dish with butter. Place flour mixture into baking dish. Place blackberries and remaining sugar in saucepan and bring to a boil. Pour fruit mixture over batter.

Bake at 400° F until golden brown.

Calories: 262
Carbohydrates: 59 g
Iron: Less than 1 mg

Cholesterol: 1 mg
Fat: 1 g
Sodium: 30 mg

Carrot-Raisin Bread

1½ cups sifted all-purpose flour

½ cup sugar

1 tsp baking powder

¼ tsp baking soda

½ tsp salt

1½ tsp ground cinnamon

¼ tsp ground allspice

1 egg, beaten

½ cup water

2 Tbsp vegetable oil

½ tsp vanilla extract

1½ cups finely shredded carrots

¼ cup chopped pecans

¼ cup golden raisins (or dried dates or dried apricots)

Preheat oven to 350° F. Lightly oil 9x5x3-inch loaf pan.

Stir together dry ingredients in large mixing bowl. Make a well in center of dry mixture.

In separate bowl, mix together remaining ingredients; add this mixture all at once to dry ingredients. Stir just enough to moisten and evenly distribute carrots.

Turn into prepared pan. Bake 50 minutes or until toothpick inserted in center comes out clean.

Cool 5 minutes in pan. Remove from pan and complete cooling on wire rack before slicing.

---

*Calories: 99	Cholesterol: 12 mg
Total fat: 3 g	Sodium: 97 mg
Saturated fat: Less than 1 g	

Mousse à la Banana

2 Tbsp low-fat (1%) milk
4 tsp sugar
1 tsp vanilla extract
1 medium banana, cut in quarters
1 cup plain low-fat yogurt
8 ¼-inch banana slices

Place milk, sugar, vanilla, and banana in blender. Process 15 seconds at high speed until smooth.

Pour mixture into a small bowl; fold in yogurt. Chill. Spoon into 4 dessert dishes; garnish each with 2 banana slices just before serving.

*Calories: 94	Cholesterol: 4 mg
Total fat: 1 g	Sodium: 47 mg
Saturated fat: 1 g	

Crunchy Pumpkin Pie

MAKES 1 9-INCH PIE—SERVING SIZE: ⅑ OF PIE

Piecrust

> 1 cup quick-cooking oats
> ¼ cup whole wheat flour
> ¼ cup ground almonds
> 2 Tbsp brown sugar
> ¼ tsp salt
> 3 Tbsp vegetable oil
> 1 Tbsp water

Pie Filling

> ¼ cup packed brown sugar
> ½ tsp ground cinnamon
> ¼ tsp ground nutmeg
> ¼ tsp salt
> 1 egg, beaten
> 4 tsp vanilla extract
> 1 cup canned pumpkin
> ⅔ cup evaporated skim milk

Preheat oven to 425° F.

Mix oats, flour, almonds, sugar, and salt together in small mixing bowl.

Blend oil and water together in measuring cup with fork or small wire whisk until emulsified.

Add oil mixture to dry ingredients and mix well. If needed, add small amount of water to hold mixture together.

Press into 9-inch pie pan and bake 8 to 10 minutes, until light brown.

Turn oven down to 350° F.

Mix sugar, cinnamon, nutmeg, and salt together in bowl.

Add eggs and vanilla and mix to blend ingredients.

Add pumpkin and milk and stir to combine.

Pour into prepared pie shell.

Bake 45 minutes or until knife inserted near center comes out clean.

---

*Calories: 177	Cholesterol: 24 mg
Total fat: 8 g	Sodium: 153 mg
Saturated fat: 1 g	

Four Play Fruit Medley

½ cantaloupe
½ honeydew melon
2 cups watermelon cubes
1 cup blueberries
2 Tbsp honey
2 Tbsp lemon juice
2 Tbsp Triple Sec orange liqueur (or orange extract)

Use melonballer to make cantaloupe and honeydew balls. Remove seeds from watermelon and cut watermelon into small cubes.

Mix fruit together in glass serving dish, reserving ½ cup of blueberries for garnish.

In small saucepan over low heat, combine honey and lemon juice; stir until blended. Blend in liqueur or orange extract. Mix thoroughly, remove from heat, and cool.

Pour sauce over fruit, cover, and refrigerate until serving time. Serve in stemmed glasses and garnish with blueberries.

Calories: 120   Fat: 1 g
Cholesterol: 0 mg

Maple-Poached Pears

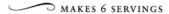

MAKES 6 SERVINGS

¼ cup raisins
¼ cup chopped nuts
¼ cup maple syrup
½ tsp lemon peel
¼ tsp ground cinnamon
3 fresh large pears, pared, halved, and cored

Preheat oven to 350° F. Combine raisins, nuts, syrup, lemon peel, and cinnamon; set aside.

Arrange pears, cut-side down, in baking dish. Cover with foil.

Bake 30 minutes or until pears are soft. Turn pears over and place spoonful of maple mixture into center of each pear. Return to oven and bake an additional 15 minutes.

Calories: 141	**Fiber:** 3 g
Fat: 3 g	**Sodium:** 12 mg
Cholesterol: 0 mg	

Peachy Berry

2 fresh peaches, sliced
2 Tbsp plain nonfat yogurt
½ cup fruit sauce
Fresh or frozen red berries, puréed
1 Tbsp packed brown sugar or honey

Arrange peach slices on 2 dessert plates. Top each with 1 tablespoon yogurt.

In 1-quart microwave-safe dish, combine berries and brown sugar. Cover and microwave on high 2 minutes or until mixture boils.

Drizzle sauce over peach slices.

---

*Calories: 103	Fiber: 3g
Percent of calories from fat: 9%	Sodium: 14 mg
Fat: 1 g	Cholesterol: 0 mg

Cupid's Quiver

1 pound medium-sized firm whole strawberries
4 ounces semisweet chocolate

Place chocolate in double boiler and cook until fully melted.

Wash strawberries, leaving stems on fruit. Pat until completely dry with paper towel.

Dip each strawberry into melted chocolate, covering lower half of berry.

Place on baking sheet lined with waxed paper. Refrigerate for at least 1 hour.

Calories: 48

Calories from fat: 18

Fat: 2 g

Saturated fat: 1.1 g

Cholesterol: 0 mg

Sodium: 0 mg

9

What's the Mind Got to Do, Got to Do with It?

How Kinsey Saved Us from Neurosis

We have been victimized by an archaic point of view. Freud sold us on all sorts of absurd sex-guilt hang-ups that slam the brakes on satisfying bedroom performance. In the not-so-distant past, the only person to whom you could talk about your sex life was a therapist. As author Richard Webster has pointed out in the introduction to *Why Freud Was Wrong: Sin, Science and Psychoanalysis*, ". . . Freud's own attitude towards some of the commonest forms of sexual behaviour, including masturbation, homosexuality and many aspects of women's sexuality, was one of distaste bordering on disgust."

As we explained in chapter 1, the sexual anatomy of the typical woman limits pleasurable sensations to a region that extends 1 to 2 inches (G-spot) into the vagina. Therefore, Freud did countless women a tremendous disservice by branding them "frigid" if they were unable to experience an orgasm during intercourse. This resulted in a therapeutic approach to sexual dysfunction that in many cases only compounded the problem.

And then along came Kinsey. The first Kinsey report published in 1948 under the title *Sexual Behavior in the Human Male,* and followed in 1950 by *Sexual Behavior in the Human Female,* contradicted the commonly held views of the time regarding sexual behavior in both men and women.

The reports were based on direct observation as well as detailed interviews, and contrary to Freudian thought, they held that "Masturbation was the most important sexual outlet for single women and the second most important sexual outlet for married women, providing 7–10 percent of their orgasms for those 16–40."

Fortunately for men, the advent of medications that treat erectile dysfunction at the physiological source of the problem has helped millions of them get back into bed. We are lagging, however, in our understanding of and approach to sexuality in women.

For many women, the issue is not so much dysfunction as dissatisfaction. *Great Food, Great Sex* is based on nutritional principles that offer readers of both sexes an easy-to-implement eating plan to foster not only more sex but also more satisfying sex through healthy meals packed with antioxidants and vitalizing NO-rich foods.

As psychologists, we recognize that there are a few things of such a nature that we'd like to bring to your attention even as you are—with great anticipation—avidly racking up grams of arginine and adding up ORAC units in your next meal.

What you are holding in your hand is the only book ever written about the care and feeding of your blood vessel endothelium—on which bedroom zip depends.

THE MIND–BODY RELATIONSHIP

> *The very problem of mind and body suggests division; I do not know of anything so disastrously affected by the habit of division as this particular theme.*
>
> —JOHN DEWEY, 1929

As simple and appealing as our plan sounds, we appreciate that having a great sex life isn't only about getting NO to reshuffle the blood flow to various organs of our body. Sex *does* begin in the mind. The mind sorts out sights, sounds, and smells and determines which of these key in to lovemaking. We are turned on by an object of sexual desire because the mind says so.

Thus, the mind mediates and modifies our behavior in accordance with biological rules. As evidenced by the wide range of sexual interests and lifestyles, these "rules" can be highly personal.

In our Western culture, reproduction is less and less related to sex and sexuality. In nature, peak sexual performance guarantees substantial contributions to the gene pool. The science of reproductive biology is still the foundation of sexuality, and it centers on brain-signaled, hormone-triggered behaviors coupled with appropriate timely changes in regional blood vessel function.

The mind sets into motion the chemical messengers to initiate the process of sexuality: Finding someone attractive triggers the ACh-NO-cGMP cascade. In fact, we are now so sophisticated that lovers may talk about there being "chemistry" between them. They're right—attraction is mediated by chemical reactions.

Knowing that the mind initiates the biochemical sequence that leads to lovemaking, we tend to blame the mind when the body fails to turn in a satisfactory (and satisfying) performance. On some occasions, that could certainly be true—thoughts and feelings can derail great sex. But more often than not, it's our physiology that lets us down. Even with the best mental intent, we can't generate an adequate supply of NO if the basic building blocks are missing. That's why, for many of us, it's high time to put a nutritional tiger back in the tank.

NOT TONIGHT DEAR—YOU'VE GIVEN ME A HEADACHE

A documented example of sexual dysfunction not being all in the mind was reported in *Annals of Internal Medicine* (Tally and Crawley, 1985). A man with severe atherosclerotic artery disease was given a nitrate patch to wear as an alternative to sublingual nitroglycerin to control his angina pain.

It was not known then that nitrates and nitroglycerine are both powerful NO donors. The patch gave him headaches, so he tried putting it on different locations on his body. When he placed it on his penis, he experienced the first erection he'd had in years. This was followed by intercourse with his wife—who reported headaches, because she was now absorbing nitrates in her vagina from his penis.

This episode could have been the key to the discovery that something in nitrates will dilate the arteries in the penis, increasing blood flow there as well as in the coronary arteries. Sadly, it did not. It was simply dismissed as an offhand "caveat" about the misuse of nitrate patches. No one seemed to comprehend that we have *one* cardiovascular system, and that blood vessels work the same way throughout the body.

ANXIETY AND SEXUAL DYSFUNCTION

Feelings of anxiety and unresolved emotional problems can contribute to performance failures . . . but performance failures can cause anxiety and emotional problems as well. It becomes a case of "chicken versus egg," when all that's really important is to experience pleasurable, satisfying sex on repeated occasions. Our food plan can help ensure that your body is prepared for the physical work of sex so that you can relax and enjoy the results.

In many cases where sex therapy fails it is because we concentrate on treating the performance anxiety when we should be looking for other causes. After all, as far as we know, Viagra does not reduce anxiety—yet it has returned countless users to very satisfactory performance.

The lasting gift that Viagra and drugs like it have given us is that they've made so many men of all ages realize that their sexual dysfunction was not all in their minds. Before Viagra, lack of performance was primarily considered a function of low or missing libido. Partners blamed themselves for being unattractive, and sex fell by the wayside. Viagra and the drugs in its class have helped men get back into bed with confidence that they could fulfill themselves and their partners. And it's accomplished with better chemistry.

GETTING BACK INTO THE SWING OF THINGS

For many Americans, regular sexual relations have become few and far between. It is easy for a sexual relationship to erode even in a good marriage because of the relentless stress and strain of everyday life. Many people value a good night's sleep more than sex, and even young couples contend they are both too tired and too busy to have sex on a regular basis. The irony is that good sex is an excellent sleep aid, as well as an effective stress reliever once you get sex back in your life.

If you are reading this book because you have gotten out of the habit of enjoying regular sexual relations, we offer the following points for your consideration and that of your partner:

- Getting back into the swing of things may require some emotional adjustments.

- Reintroducing romance and sex in a relationship from which they have been missing for some time may seem awkward at first.

- Lovemaking does not have to be spontaneous each time to be enjoyable; nor must it invariably lead to intercourse. Don't be afraid to try a morning "quickie" or giving each other a soothing massage. You don't need a perfect moment to make love, but you do need to be understanding and accepting of each other.

For many, our diet plan will add zest and help bring you to an even more enjoyable level of lovemaking. But if you are trying to reintroduce sexual activity when it has been lacking for some time, remember: Just as with restarting any type of physical activity, it helps to start slow and build up. The injured "Weekend Warrior" is a common visitor to many orthopedic practices. This is usually a middle-aged man who decides to go for a long run or play a hard game of singles tennis after he has been physically sedentary for a number of years.

Many couples who truly love each other have an otherwise stable and satisfying relationship though there may be very little or no satisfying sex. While it may be frustrating to one or both partners, it has not become a reason for them to separate. Reintroducing sex in a relationship where it may have been absent for some time may require counseling from a competent family therapist.

Dwindling sex may happen for a number of reasons, including health concerns. For women, hormonal changes may have made lovemaking increasingly uncomfortable. Many women's health magazines provide competent advice on vaginal lubrication that can make a world of difference. Vaginal lubricants can help ease the way back into comfortable lovemaking. But not all lubricants are created equal. Beware of petroleum-based formulations as these can harbor bacteria in the vagina and lead to infection as well as damage to latex condoms. Most pharmacies now offer a variety of water-based lubricants in the feminine product section.

Men may become gradually less inclined to lovemaking with their partner if it is clearly uncomfortable for her. Sex may at first be hurried, and that causes additional problems; it does not allow sufficient foreplay time for adequate lubrication. Take your time and don't be concerned about having intercourse every time you go to bed together.

In addition, with increasing age, lovers may ultimately succumb to the constant barrage of media messages that sex is only for the young. Our culture has bought into the myth that sexuality inevitably fades away with age. Today's "macho stud" is tomorrow's "dirty old man."

The best thing that has happened to the aging population in the United States is the increasing number of studies and media reports that find that sex is a legitimate concern for the mature population: A hitherto unknown—and vast—number of our maturing Americans are doing it regularly—well into their eighties and, for the most part, with gusto. So said the National Counsel on the Aging in a 1998 report titled "Healthy Sexuality and Vital Aging." Great sex is the gift that keeps on giving, and age is not a barrier.

IT IS NEVER TOO LATE TO BECOME WHAT YOU MIGHT
HAVE BEEN. —GEORGE ELIOT

Habits, good or bad, helpful or harmful, are the basis of most human behaviors: The best way to predict what you will do tomorrow is to see what you did yesterday. And so it is for food. We reach for foods we are in the habit of eating, and we are in the habit of eating foods that are at hand . . . because we are in the habit of purchasing them.

To successfully adopt our food plan, you have to think outside of the doughnut box and dare to shop, prepare meals, and eat more mindfully. To change habits, particularly ingrained ones such as skipping breakfast, you need to consciously examine your behavior and strategize to modify it. Modest, cumulative changes have the best chance of becoming a permanent feature of your behavioral repertoire. If you have not eaten breakfast for the past twenty years, you may need to gradually shift the timing of your meals so that you actually feel hungry when you wake up. Whenever possible, try to cue into your own body clock rather than relying on a fixed schedule for meals. Eating when you are really hungry makes even the simplest food taste better.

The same goes for romance: It is so easy to get out of the habit of being romantic, and yet, with improving sexual vitality, reintroducing romance where it has been waning may make a world of difference to the quality of your life and that of your partner's. If you take the trouble to improve your performance, take the trouble to properly set the stage.

If you have gotten out of the habit of holding hands, try going to a movie together, where you can snuggle. Try bringing flowers home without a specific occasion—yes, men do appreciate the gesture. Leave a love note on the bathroom mirror.

Most of all, pay attention to each other. Preparing a great meal together makes for wonderful foreplay. Set a table with the care you would expect in a restaurant, put on some nice music, and enjoy the time together. And this does not presume there are no children in the picture: Providing affectionate role models for your children will help them build successful relationships as they grow up.

The foods that make up the Great Food, Great Sex plan are healthy choices for every member of the family, so don't worry about having to cook separate meals for the kids.

Finally, don't let hours spent in front of the television sap your desire. Too many of us waste precious time dozing in front of the tube. A short after-dinner walk together is a great way to get your juices flowing. Get off the couch and into bed!

Bibliography

Abe, Y., El-Masri. B., Kimball, K. T., Pownall, H., Reilly, C. F., Osmundsen, K., Smith, C. W., & Ballantyne, C. M. (1998): Soluble cell adhesion molecules in hypertriglyceridemia and potential significance on monocyte adhesion. *Arteriosclerosis, Thrombosis & Vascular Biology,* 18, 723–731.

Adamson, G. E., Lazarus, S. A., Mitchell, A. E., Prior, R. L., Cao, G., Jacobs, P. H., Kremers, B. G., Hammerstone, J. F., Rucker, R. B., Ritter, K. A., & Schmitz, H. H. (1999): HPLC method for the quantification of procyanidins in cocoa and chocolate samples and correlation to total antioxidant capacity. *J. Agric. Food. Chem.,* 47, 4184–4188.

Agarwal, C., Sharma, Y., Zhao, J., & Agarwal, R. (2000): A polyphenolic fraction from grape seeds causes irreversible growth inhibition of breast carcinoma MDA-MB468 cells by inhibiting mitogen-activated protein kinases activation and inducing G1 arrest and differentiation. *Clinical Cancer Research*, 6, 2921–2930.

Agarwal, C., Singh, R. P., & Agarwal, R. (2002): Grape seed extract induces apoptotic death of human prostate carcinoma DU 145 cells via caspaces activation accompanied by dissipation of mitochondrial membrane potential and cytochrome c release. *Carcinogenesis*, 23, 1867–1876.

Ahlqwist, M., Bengtsson, C., Lapidus, L., Gergdahl, I. A., & Schutz, A. (1999): Serum mercury concentration in relation to survival, symptoms, and diseases: results from the prospective population study of women in Gothenburg, Sweden. *Acta Odontologica Scandinavica,* 57, 168–174.

Albert, C. M., Gaziano, J. M., Willett, W. C., & Manson, J. E. (2002): Nut consumption and decreased risk of sudden cardiac death in the Physicians' Health Study. *Archives of Internal Medicine*, 162, 1382–1387.

Aldini, G., Carini, M., Piccoli, A., Rossoni, G., & Facino, R. M. (2003): Procyanidins from grape seeds protect endothelial cells from peroxynitrite damage and enhance endothelium-dependent relaxation of human artery: new evidence for cardio-protection. *Life Sciences*, 73, 2883–2898.

Allen, M. (1987): A holistic view of sexuality. *Holistic Nursing Practice*, 1, 4.

Alper, C. M., & Matte, R. D. (2002): Effects of chronic peanut consumption on energy balance and hedonics. *Int. J. Obes. & Rel. Disord.*, 26, 1129–1137.

Althof, S. E., Cort, E. W., Levine, S. B., Levine, F., Burnett, A. L., McVary, K., Stecher, V., & Seftel, A. D. (1999): EDITS: Development of questionnaires for evaluating sat-isfaction with treatments for erectile dysfunction. *Urology*, 53, 793–799.

Artaud-Wild, S. M., Connor, S. L., Sexton, G., & Connor, W. E. (1993): Differences in coronary mortality can be explained by differences in cholesterol and saturated fat intakes in 40 countries but not in France and Finland: a paradox. *Circulation*, 88, 2771–2779.

Ascherio, A., Rimm, E. B., Stampfer, M. J., Giovannucci, E. L., & Willett, W. C. (1995): Dietary intake of marine n-3 fatty acids, fish intake, and the risk of coro-nary disease among men. *New England Journal of Medicine*, 332, 977–982.

Bagchi, D., Bagchi, M., Stohs, S. J., Das, D. K., Ray, S. D., Kuszynsk, C. A., Joshi, S. S., & Prues, H. G. (2000): Free radicals and grape seed proanthocyanidin extract: im-portance in human health and disease prevention. *Toxicology*, 148, 187–197.

Bagchi, D., Bagchi, M., Stohs, S., Ray, S. D., Sen, C. K., & Preuss, H. G. (2002): Cellu-lar protection with proanthocyanidins derived from grape seeds. *Annals of the New York Academy of Science*, 957, 260–270.

Balch, J. F. (1998): *The Super Antioxidants*. New York: M. Evans & Co.

Balch, J. F., & Balch, P. A. (1997): *Prescription for Nutritional Healing*. 2nd ed. Garden City Park, NY: Avery Publishing.

Bankroft, J. (1989): Assessing people with sexual problems. In *Human Sexuality and Its Problems*. Edinburgh: Churchill Livingstone, 412–455.

Barksdale, J. D., & Gardner, S. F. (1999): The impact of first-line antihypertensive drugs on erectile dysfunction. *Pharmacotherapy*, 19, 573–581.

Basson, R. (2001): Female sexual response: the role of drugs in the management of sex-ual dysfunction. *Obstetrics & Gynecology*, 98, 350–353.

Basson, R., Berman, J., Burnett, A., Derogatis, L., Ferguson, D., Fourcroy, J., Gol-stein, I., Graziottin, A., Heiman, J., Laan, E., Leiblum, S., Padma-Nathan, H., Rosen, R., Segraves, K., Segraves, R. T., Shabsigh, R., Sipski, M., Wagner, G., & Whipple, B. (2000): Report of the international consensus development conference on female sexual dysfunction: definitions and classifications. *Journal of Urology*, 163, 888–893.

Bastianetto, S., & Quirion, R. (2002): Natural extracts as possible protective agents of brain aging. *Neurobiology of Aging*, 23, 891–897.

Belalcazar, L. M., & Ballantyne, C. M. (1998): Defining specific goals of therapy in treating dyslipidemia in the patient with low high-density lipoprotein cholesterol. *Progress in Cardiovascular Diseases*, 41, 151–174.

Berman, J. R, & Bassuk, J. (2002): Physiology and pathophysiology of female sexual function and dysfunction. *World Journal of Urology*, 20, 111–118.

Berman, J. R., Berman, L. A., Werbin, T. J., & Golstein, I. (1999): Female sexual dysfunction: anatomy, physiology, evaluation and treatment options. *Curr Opin Urol.*, 9, 563–568. Review.

Bernardo, A. (2001): Sexuality in patients with coronary disease and heart failure. *Herz* (heart), 26, 353–359.

Bhat, K. P. L., Kosmeder, J. W. 2nd, & Pessuto, J. M. (2001): Biological effects of resveratrol. *Antioxidants & Redox Signaling*, 3, 1041–1064.

Bistrian, B. R. (2004): Practical recommendations for immune-enhancing diets. *Journal of Nutrition*, 134, 2868S.

Bitsch, R., Netzel, M., Frank, T., Strass, G., & Bitsch, I. (2004): Bioavailability and bio-kinetics of anthocyanins from red grape juice and red wine. *Journal of Biomedicine & Biotechnology*, 5, 293–298.

Blanchflower, D. G., & Oswald, A. J. (2004): Money, sex and happiness: an empirical study. *Scandinavian Journal of Economics* (special issue), 106, 393–415.

Blomhoff, R. (2005): Dietary antioxidants and cardiovascular disease. *Current Opinion in Lipidology*, 16, 47–54.

Blum, A., & Miller, H. (1999): The effects of L-arginine on atherosclerosis and heart disease. *International Journal of Cardiovascular Interventions*, 2, 97–100.

Blumentals, W. A., Gomez-Caminero, A., Joo, S., & Vannappagari, V. (2004): Should erectile dysfunction be considered as a marker for acute myocardial infarction? Results from a retrospective study. *Aging Male*, 6, 217–221.

Bode-Boger, S. M., Muke, J., Surdacki, A., Brabant, G., Boger, R. H., & Frolich, J. C. (2003): Oral L-arginine improves endothelial function in healthy individuals older than 70 years. *Vascular Medicine*, 8, 77–81.

Bosetti, C., La Vecchia, C., Talamini, R., Simonato, L., Zambon, P., Negri, E., Trichopoulos, D., Lagiou, P., Bardini, R., & Franceschi, S. (2000): Food groups and risk factors of squamous cell esophageal cancer in northern Italy. *International Journal of Cancer*, 87, 289–294.

Braverman, E. R., & Pfeiffer, C. C. (1987): *The Healing Nutrients Within*. New Caanan, CT: Keats Publishing, Inc.

Brecker, E. (1984): *Love, Sex, and Aging: A Consumer's Union Report*. Boston: Little Brown.

Bronte, V., Kasic, T., Gri, G., Gallana, K., Borsellino, G., Marigo, I., Battistini, L., Iafrate, M., Prayer-Galetti, T., Pagano, F., & Viola, A. (2005): Boosting antitumor responses of T lymphocytes infiltrating human prostate cancers. *Journal of Experimental Medicine*, 18, 201, 1257–1268. (Epub)

Brouillard, R., George, F., & Fougerousse, A. (1997): Polyphenols produced during red wine aging. *Biofactors*, 6, 403–410.

Bruder, J. L., Hsieh, T. C., Lerea, K. M., Olson, S. C., & Wu, J. M. (2001): Induced cytoskeletal changes in bovine pulmonary artery endothelial cells by resveratrol and the accompanying modified response to arterial shear stress. *BMC Cell Biology*, 2, 1.

Buck, A. C. (2004): Is there a scientific basis for the therapeutic effects of serenoa repens in benign prostatic hyperplasia? Mechanisms of action. *Journal of Urology*, 172, 1792–1799.

Burnett, A. L. (1995): Nitric oxide control of lower genitourinary tract functions: a review. *Urology*, 45, 1071–1083.

Burnett, A. L., Calvin, D. C., Silver, R. I., Peppas, D. S., & Docimo, S. G. (1997): Immunohistochemical description of nitric oxide synthase isoforms in human clitoris. *Journal of Urology*, 158, 75–78.

Burnett, A. L., Lowenstein, C. J., Bredt, D. S., Chang, T. S. K., & Snyder, S. H. (1992): Nitric oxide: a physiologic mediator of penile erection. *Science*, 257, 401–403.

Burnett, A. L., Tillman, S. L., Chang, T. S. K., Epstein, J. I., Lowenstein, C. J., Bredt, D. S., Snyder, S. H., & Walsh, P. C. (1993): Immunohistochemical localization of nitric oxide synthase in the autonomic nervous innervation of the human penis. *Journal of Urology*, 150, 73–76.

Camargo, C. A., Jr. (1989): Moderate alcohol consumption and stroke: the epidemiologic evidence. *Stroke*, 29, 1611–1626.

Campbell, J. K., Canene-Adams, K., Lindshield, B. L., Boileau, T. W., Clinton, S. K., & Erdman, J. W., Jr. (2004): Tomato phytochemicals and prostate cancer. *Journal of Nutrition*, 134, 3486S–3492S.

Canoy, D., Wareham, N., Welch, A., Bingham, S., Luben, R., Day, N., & Khaw, K. T. (2005): Plasma ascorbic acid concentrations and fat distribution in 19,068 British men and women in the European Prospective Investigation into Cancer and Nutrition Norfolk cohort study. *Am. J. Clin. Nutr.*, 82, 1203–1209.

Cao, G., Alessio, H. M., & Cutler, R. G. (1993): Oxygen-radical absorbance capacity assay of antioxidants. *Free Radical Biology & Medicine*, 14, 303–311.

Cao, G., Russell, R. M., Lischner, N., & Prior, L. (1998): Serum antioxidant capacity is increased by consumption of strawberries, spinach, red wine or vitamin C in elderly women. *Journal of Nutrition*, 128, 2383–2390.

Carter, A. M. (2005): Inflammation, thrombosis and acute coronary syndromes. *Diab. Vasc. Dis. Res.*, 2, 113–121. Review.

Caruso, D., Berra, B., Giavarini, F., Cortesi, N., Fedeli, E., & Galli, G. (1999): Effect of virgin olive oil phenolic compounds on in vitro oxidation of human low density lipoproteins. *Nutrition, Metabolism & Cardiovascular Diseases*, 9, 102–107.

Catapano, A. L. (1997): Antioxidant effect of flavonoids. *Angiology*, 48, 39–44.

Chaitlin, M. D. (2004): Erectile dysfunction: the earliest sign of generalized vascular disease? *Journal of the American College of Cardiology*, 43, 185–186.

Chin, J. P., & Dart, A. M. (1995): How do fish oils affect vascular function? *Clinical Experimental Pharmacology & Physiology*, 22, 71–81.

Chung, W. S., Sohn, J. H., & Park, Y. Y. (1999): Is obesity an underlying factor in erectile dysfunction? *European Urology*, 36, 68–70.

Clarkson, P., Adams, M. R., Powe, A. J., Donald, A. E., McCredie, R., Robinson, J., McCarthy, S. N., Keech, A., Celermajer, D. S., & Deanfield, J. E. (1996): Oral L-arginine improves endothelium-dependent dilation in hypercholesterolemic young adults. *Journal of Clinical Investigation*, 97, 1989–1994.

Clifton, P. M. (2004): Effect of grape extract and quercetin on cardiovascular and endothelial parameters in high-risk subjects. *Journal of Biomedicine & Biotechnology*, 5, 272–278.

Coe, S. D., & Coe, M. D. (1996): *The True History of Chocolate*. New York: Thames and Hudson, 1996.

Connell, K., Guess, M. K., Bleustein, C. B., Powers, K., Lazarou, G., Mikhail, M., & Melman, A. (2005): Effects of age, menopause, and comorbidities on neurological function of the female genitalia. *International Journal of Impotence Research*, 17, 63–70.

Cooray, H. C., Janvilisri, T., van Veen, H. W., Hladky, S. B., & Barrand, M. A. (2004): Interaction of breast cancer resistance protein with plant polyphenols. *Biochemistry & Biophysics Research Communication*, 317, 268–275.

Corti, M. C., Gurlanik, J. M., & Bilato, C. (1996): Coronary heart disease risk factors in older persons. *Aging*, 2, 75–89.

Criqui, N. M. (1998): Do known cardiovascular risk factors mediate the effect of alcohol on cardiovascular disease? *Novartis Foundation Symposium*, 216, 159–167; discussion 167–172.

Dai, Z., Zhu, H. Q., Jiang, D. J., Jiang, J. L., Deng, H. W., & Li, Y. J. (2004): 17-Beta-estradiol preserves endothelial function by reduction of the endogenous nitric oxide synthase inhibitor level. *International Journal of Cardiology*, 96, 223–227.

D'Amati, G., di Gioia, C. R., Bologna, M., Giordano, D., Giorgi, M., Dolci, S., & Jannini, E. A. (2002): Type 5 phosphodiesterase expression in human vagina. *Urology*, 60, 191–195.

Das, D. K., Sato, M., Ray, P. S., Maulik, G., Engelman, R. M., Bertelli, A. A., & Bertelli, A. (1999): Cardioprotection of red wine: role of polyphenolic antioxidants. *Drugs & Experimental & Clinical Research*, 25, 115–120.

Dash, E. (2004): Sex may be happiness, but wealth isn't sexiness. *The New York Times—Ideas & Trends*, Sunday, July 11.

Davey Smith, G., Frankel, S., & Yarnell, J. (1997): Sex and death: are they related? Findings from the Caerphilly Cohort Study. *British Medical Journal*, 315, 1641–1644.

de Gaetano, G., & Cerletti, C. (2001): Wine and cardiovascular disease. *Nutrition, Metabolism & Cardiovascular Diseases*, 11(4 Suppl), 47–50.

Deiana, M., Aruomo, O. I., Bianchi, M. L., Spencer, J. P., Kaur, H., Halliwell, B., Aeschbach, R., Banni, S., Dessi, M. A., & Corongiu, F. P. (1999): Inhibition of peroxynitrite dependent DNA base modification and tyrosine nitration by the extra virgin oil–derived antioxidant hydroxytyrosol. *Free Radical Biology & Medicine*, 26, 762–769.

Della Chiesa, A., Pfiffner, D., Meier, B., & Hess, O. (2003): Sexual activity in hypertensive men. *Journal of Human Hypertension*, 17, 515–521.

de Lorgeril, K., Salen, P., Martin, J. L., Monjaud, I., Delaye, J., & Mamelle, N. (1999): Mediterranean diet, traditional risk factors, and the rate of cardiovascular complications after myocardial infarction: final report of the Lyon Diet Heart Study. *Circulation*, 99, 779–785.

de Lorimier, A. A. (2000): Alcohol, wine, and health. *American Journal of Surgery*, 180, 357–361.

Demrow, H. S., Slane, P. R., & Folts, J. D. (1995): Administration of wine and grape juice inhibits in vivo platelet activity and thrombosis in stenosed canine coronary arteries. *Circulation*, 91, 1182–1188.

Department of Health and Human Services, US Food and Drug Administration: Substances affirmed as generally recognized as safe: menhaden oil. *Federal Register*. June 5, 1997. Vol. 62, No. 108: 30751–30757. 21 CFR Part 184. Docket No. 86G-0289. Available at: http://frwebgate.access.gpo.gov/cgi-bin/getdoc.cgi?db name=1997_register&docid=fr05jn97-5. Accessed October 3, 2002.

Derby, C. A., Mohr, B. A., Goldstein, I., Feldman, H. A., Johannes, C. B., & McKinlay, J. B. (2000): Modifiable risk factors and erectile dysfunction: can lifestyle changes modify risk? *Urology*, 56, 302–306.

Dewey, J. (1929): *Experience and Nature*. New York: Dover.

Dizdaroglu, M., Jaruga, P., Birincioglu, M., & Rodriguez, H. (2002): Free radical–induced damage to DNA: mechanisms and measurement. *Free Radical Biology & Medicine*, 32, 1102–1115.

Durak, I., Yalcin, S., Kacmaz, M., Cimen, M. Y., Buyukkocak, S., Avci, A., & Ozturk, H. S. (1999): High-temperature effects on antioxidant systems and toxic product formation in nutritional oils. *Journal of Toxicology & Environmental Health*, 57, 585–589.

Dvorkin, L., & Song, K. Y. (2002): Herbs for benign prostatic hyperplasia. *Annals of Pharmacotherapy*, 36, 1443–1452.

Ebrahim, S., May, M., Ben Shlomo, Y., McCarron, P., Frankel, S., Yarnell, J., & Davey Smith, G. (2002): Sexual intercourse and risk of ischaemic stroke and coronary heart disease: the Caerphilly study. *Journal of Epidemiology & Community Health*, 56, 99–102.

Elder, J., & Braver, Y. (2003): Disease management project: female sexual dysfunction. www.clevelandclinicmeded.com/diseasemanagement/women/sex_dysfunction/sex_dysfunction.htm.

Eng, E. T., Ye, J., Williams, D., Phung, S., Moore, R. E., Young, M. K., Gruntmanis, U., Braunstein, G., Chen, S. (2003): Suppression of estrogen biosynthesis by procyanidin dimers in red wine and grape seeds. *Cancer Research*, 63, 8516–8522.

European Prospective Investigation on Diet and Cancer (EPIC) (1999): Consumption patterns and the principal sources of lipids and fatty acids in the Spanish cohort of the European Prospective Investigation on Diet and Cancer (EPIC). The EPIC Group in Spain. *Medica Clinica* (Barcelona), 112, 125–132.

Farinaro, E., Panico, S., & Jossa, F. (1992): Diet and cardiovascular risk in women in Italy. *Annali Dell'Istituto Superiore di Sanita*, 28, 349–353.

Farnham, A. (2003): Is sex necessary? www.Forbes.com.

Feinman, L., & Lieber, C. S. (1999): Ethanol and lipid metabolism. *American Journal of Clinical Nutrition*, 70, 791–792.

Fisher, N. D., Hughes, M., Gerhard-Herman, M., & Hollenberg, N. K. (2003): Flavonol-rich cocoa induces nitric-oxide-dependent vasodilation in healthy humans. *Journal of Hypertension*, 21, 2281–2286.

Fito, M., Covas, M. I., Lamuela-Raventos, R. M., Vila, J., Torrents, L., de la Torre, C., & Marrugat, J. (2000): Protective effect of olive oil and its phenolic compounds against low density lipoprotein oxidation. *Lipids*, 35, 633–638.

Fitzpatrick, D. F., Bing, B., & Rohdewald, P. (1998): Endothelium-dependent vascular effects of pycnogenol. *Journal of Cardiovascular Pharmacology*, 32, 509–515.

Franceschi, S., Favero, A., Conti, E., Talamini, R., Volpe, R., Negri, E., Barzan, L., & La Vecchia, C. (1999): Food groups, oils and butter, and cancer of the oral cavity and pharynx. *British Journal of Cancer,* 80, 614–620.

Francis, G., Kerem, Z., Makkar, H. P., & Becker, K. (2002): The biological action of saponins in animal system: a review. *British Journal of Nutrition,* 88, 587–605.

Fraser, G. E. (1999): Nut consumption, lipids, and risk of a coronary event. *Clinical Cardiology,* 22 (III Suppl.), S11–S15.

Fraser, G. E., Sabate, J., Beeson, W. L., Strahan, T. M. (1992): A possible protective effect of nut consumption on risk of coronary heart disease: The Adventist Health Study. *Archives of Internal Medicine,* 152, 1416–1424.

Freedman, J. E., Parker, C., 3rd, Li, L., Perlman, J. A., Ivanov, V., Deak, L. R., Iafrati, M. D., & Folts, J. D. (2001): Select flavonoids and whole juice from purple grapes inhibit platelet function and enhance nitric oxide release. *Circulation,* 103, 2782–2798.

Fried, R., & Merrel, W. C., with Thornton, J. (1999): *The Arginine Solution.* New York: Warner Books, Inc.

Friedman, T. L. (2000): *The Lexus and the Olive Tree.* New York: Farrar Strauss & Giroux.

Fuentes, F., Lopez-Miranda, J., Sanchez, E., Sanchez, F., Paez, J., Paz-Rojas, E., Marin, C., Gomez, P., Jimenez-Pereperez, J., Ordovas, J. M., & Perez-Jimenez, F. (2002): Mediterranean and low-fat diets improve endothelial function in hypercholesterolemic men. *Annals of Internal Medicine,* 134, 1115–1119.

Fung, M. M., Bettencourt, R., & Barrett-Connor, E. (2004): Heart risk factors predict erectile dysfunction 25 years later: the Rancho Bernardo Study. *Journal of the American College of Cardiology,* 43, 1405–1411.

Furchgott, R. F. (1996): The discovery of endothelium-derived relaxing factor and its importance in the identification of nitric oxide. *Journal of the American Medical Association,* 276, 1186–1188.

Furchgott, R. F., & Zawadzki, J. V. (1990): The obligatory role of endothelial cells in the relaxation of arterial smooth muscle by acetylcholine. *Nature,* 288, 373–376.

Gallup, G. G., Jr., Burch, R. L., & Platek, S. M. (2002): Does semen have antidepressant properties? *Archives of Sexual Behavior,* 31, 289–293.

Gerra, A., Feldl, F., & Koletzko, B. (2001): Fatty acid composition of plasma lipids in healthy Portuguese children: is the Mediterranean diet disappearing? *Annals of Nutrition & Metabolism,* 45, 78–81.

Ginsberg, H., Olefsky, J., Farquhar., J. W., & Reaven, G. M. (1974): Moderate ethanol ingestion and plasma triglyceride levels: a study in normal and hypertriglyceridemic persons. *Annals of Internal Medicine,* 80, 143–149.

Giovanni, S., Staface, E., Modesti, D., Coni, E., Cantafora, A., De Vincenzi, M., Malorni, W., & Masella, R. (1999): Tyrosol, the major olive oil biophenol, protects against oxidized-LDL-induced injury in Caco-2 cells. *Journal of Nutrition,* 129, 1269–1277.

Gjonka, A., & Bobak, M. (1998): Albanian paradox: another example of protective effect of Mediterranean lifestyle? *Lancet,* 350, 1815–1817.

Goldberg, I. J., Mosca, L., Piano, M. R., & Fisher, E. A. (2001): Wine and your heart. *Circulation*, 103, 472–477.

Goldberg, J., Flowerdew, J., Smith, E., Brody, J. A., & Tsao, M. O. M. (1988): Factors associated with age-related macular degeneration: an analysis of data from the First National Health and Nutrition Examination Survey. *American Journal of Epidemiology*, 128, 700–710.

Goldstein, I., & Berman, J. R. (1998): Vasculogenic female sexual dysfunction: vaginal engorgement and clitoral erectile insufficiency syndromes. *International Journal of Impotence Research*, 10 (2 Suppl), S84–S90.

Golikov, P. P., & Nikolaeva, N. (2004): Analysis of nitrites and nitrates (Unox) in urine. *Klinicheskaia Laboratornaia Diagnostika*, Jan., 13–15.

Gonzales de Mejia, E. (2003): The chemoprotector effects of tea components. *Archives of Latinoamerican Nutrition*, 53, 111–118.

Gragasin, F. S., Michelakis, E. D., Hogan, A., Moudgil, R., Hashimoto, K., Wu, X., Bonnett, S., Haromy, A., & Archer, S. L. (2004): The neurovascular mechanism of clitoral erection: nitric oxide and cGMP-stimulated activation of BKca channels. *Federation of American Societies for Experimental Biology Journal*, 18, 1382–1391.

Grassi, D., Necozione, S., Lippi, C., Croce, G., Valeri, L., Pasqualetti, P., Desideri, G., Blumberg, J. B., & Ferri, C. (2005): Cocoa reduces blood pressure and insulin resistance and improves endothelium-dependent vasodilation in hypertensives. *Hypertension*, 46, 398–405. Epub July 18, 2005.

Greco, L., Musmarra, F., Franzese, C., & Auricchio, S. (1998): Early childhood feeding practices in southern Italy: is the Mediterranean diet becoming obsolete? Study of 450 children aged 6–32 months in Campania, Italy. *Acta Paediatrica*, 87, 250–260.

Grimsgaard, S., Bonaa, K. H., Hansen, J. B., & Nordoy, A. (1997): Highly purified eicosapentaenoic acid and docosahexaenoic acid in humans have similar triacylglycerol-lowering effects but divergent effects on serum fatty acids. *American Journal of Clinical Nutrition*. 66, 649–659.

Gronbaek, M., Deis, A., Sorensen, T. I., Becker, U., Schnohr, P., & Jensen, G. (1995): Mortality associated with moderate intakes of wine, beer, or spirits. *British Medical Journal*, 310, 1165–1169.

Harats, D., Chevion, S., Nahir, M., Norman, Y., Sagee, O., & Berry, E. M. (1998): Citrus fruit supplementation reduces lipoprotein oxidation in young men ingesting a diet high in saturated fat: presumptive evidence for an interaction between vitamin C and E in vivo. *American Journal of Clinical Nutrition*, 67, 240–245.

Harris, W. S. (1997): Fatty acids and serum lipoproteins: human studies. *American Journal of Clinical Nutrition*, 65, S1645–S1654.

Harris, W. S., Rambjor, G. S., Windsor, S. L., & Diedrich, D. (1997): N-3 fatty acids and urinary excretion of nitric oxide metabolites in humans. *American Journal of Clinical Nutrition*, 65, 459–464.

Hatzichristou, D., Hatzimouratidis, K., Bekas, M., Apostolidis, A., Tzotzis, V., & Yannakoyorgos, K. (2002): Diagnostic steps in evaluation of patients with erectile dysfunction. *Journal of Urology*, 168, 615–620.

Haywood, R., Wardman, P., Sanders, R., & Linge, C. (2003): Sunscreens inadequately protect against ultraviolet-A-induced free radicals in skin: implications for skin aging and melanoma. *Journal of Investigative Dermatology*, 121, 862–868.

Henning, S. M., Fajardo-Lira, C., Lee, H. W., Youssefian, A. A., Go, V. L., & Heber, D. (2003): Catechin content of 18 teas and a green tea extract supplement correlates with antioxidant capacity. *Nutrition & Cancer*, 45, 226–235.

Herron, K. J., Vega-Lopez, S., Conde, K., Ramjiganesh, T., Roy, S., Shachter, N., & Fernandez, M. L. (2002): Pre-menopausal women classified as hyper-responders do not alter their LDL/HDL ratio following a high dietary cholesterol challenge. *Journal of the American College of Nutrition*, 21, 250–258.

Herron, K. L., Vega-Lopez, S., Ramjiganesh, T., Conde, K., Shachter, N., & Fernandez, M. L. (2002): Men classified as hypo- or hyper-responders to a dietary cholesterol challenge exhibit differences in lipoprotein metabolism. *Journal of Nutrition*, 133, 1036–1042.

Hiipakka, R. A., Zhang, H. Z., Dai, W., Dai, Q., & Lioao, S. (2002): Structure-activity relationship for inhibition of human 5 alpha-reductase by polyphenols. *Biochemical Pharmacology*, 63, 1165–1176.

Hilz, M. J., & Marthol, H. (2003): Erectile dysfunction—value of neurophysiologic diagnostic procedures. *Urologe Ausgabe A*, 42, 1345–1350.

Hilz, M. J., & Marthol, H. (2004): Female sexual function: a systematic overview of classification, pathophysiology, diagnosis and treatment. *Fortschritte der Neurolgie-Psychiatrie*, 72, 121–135.

Hooi, J. D., Kester, A. D., Stoffers, H. E., Rinkens, P. E., Knottnerus, J. A., & van Rees, J. W. (2004): Asymptomatic peripheral arterial occlusive disease predicted cardiovascular morbidity and mortality in a 7-year follow-up study. *Journal of Clinical Epidemiology*, 57, 294–300.

Hoyle, C. H., Stones, R. W., Robson, T., Whitley, K., & Burnstock, G. (1996): Innervation of vasculature and microvasculature of the human vagina by NOS and neuropeptide-containing nerves. *Journal of Anatomy*, 188 (Pt 3), 633–644.

Hu, F. B., Bronner, L., Willett, W. C., Stampfer, M. J., Rexrode, K. M., Albert, C. M., Hunter, D., & Manson, J. E. (2002): Fish and omega-3 fatty acid intake and risk of coronary heart disease in women. *Journal of the American Medical Association*, 287,1815–1821.

Hu, F. B., Stampfer, M. J., Manson, J. E., Rimm, E. B., Colditz, G. A., Rosner, B. A., Hennekens, C. H., & Willett, W. C. (1997): Dietary fat intake and the risk of coronary heart disease in women. *New England Journal of Medicine*, 337, 1491–1499.

Hu, F. B., Stampfer, M. J., Manson, J. E., Rimm, E. B., Colditz, G. A., Rosner, B. A., Speizer, F. E., Hennekens, C. H., & Willett, W. C. (1998): Frequent nut consumption and risk of coronary heart disease in women: prospective cohort study. *British Medical Journal*, 317, 1341–1345.

Hu, F. B., Stampfer, M. J., Rimm, E. B., Manson, J. E., Ascherio, A., Colditz, G. A., Rosner, B. A., Spiegelman, D., Speizer, F. E., Sacks, F. M., Hennekens, C. H., & Willett, W. C. (1999): A prospective study of egg consumption and risk of cardiovascular disease in men and women. *Journal of the American Medical Association*, 281, 1387–1394.

Huertas, J. R., Martinez-Velasco, E., Ibanez, S., Lopez-Frias, M., Ochoa, J. J., Quiles, J., Parenti Castelli, G., Mataix, J., & Lenaz, G. (1999): Virgin olive oil and coenzyme Q10 protect heart mitochondria from peroxidative damage during aging. *Biofactors*, 9, 337–343.

Hung, L. M., Chen, J. K., Huang, S. S., Lee, R. S., & Su, M. J. (2000): Cardioprotective effect of resveratrol, a natural antioxidant derived from grapes. *Cardiovascular Research*, 47, 349–355.

Imbimbo, C., Gentile, V., Palmieri, A., Longo, N., Fusco, F., Granata, A. M., Verze, P., & Mirone, V. (2003): Female sexual dysfunction: an update on physiopathology. *Journal of Endocrinological Investigation*, 26, 102–104.

Institute of Medicine (IOM) (2002): *Dietary Reference Intakes for Energy and Macronutrients*. Washington, DC: National Academy Press.

Ipatova, O. M., Prozorovskaia, N. N., Baranova, V. S., & Guseva, D. A. (2004): Biological activity of linseed oil as a source of omega-3 alpha-linoleic acid. *Biomeditsinskaia khimiia*, 50, 25–43.

Isaksson, M., & Bruze, M. (1999): Occupational allergic contact dermatitis from olive oil in a masseur. *Journal of the American Academy of Dermatology*, 41, 312–315.

Jacob, R. A., Spinozzi, G. M., Simon, V. A., Kelley, D. S., Priorm, R. L., Hess-Pierce, B., & Kader, A. A. (2003): Consumption of cherries lowers plasma urate in healthy women. *Journal of Nutrition*, 133, 1826–1829.

Jacobsen, F. M. (1992): Fluoxetine-induced sexual dysfunction and an open trial of yohimbine. *Journal of Clinical Psychiatry*, 53, 119–122.

JAMA Patient Page (1999). Silence about sexual problems can hurt relationships. *Journal of the American Medical Association*, 281, 6, 584.

Jenkins, D. J., Kendall, C. W., Marchie, A., Faulkner, D. A., Wong, J. M., de Souza, R., Emam, A., Parker, T. L., Vidgen, E., Lapsley, K. G., Trautwein, E. A., Josse, R. G., Leiter, L. A., & Connelly, P. W. (2003): Effects of a dietary portfolio of cholesterol-lowering foods vs lovastatin on serum lipids and C-reactive protein. *Journal of the American Medical Association*, 290, 502–510.

Jenkins, D. J., Kendall, C. W., Marchie, A., Parker, T. L., Connelly, P. W., Qian, W., Haight, J. S., Faulkner, D., Vidgen, E., Lapsley, K. G., & Spiller, G. A. (2002): Dose response of almonds on coronary heart disease risk factors: blood lipids, oxidized low-density lipoproteins, lipoproteins(a), homocysteine, and pulmonary nitric oxide: a randomized, controlled, crossover trial. *Circulation*, 106, 1327–1332.

Jia, L., Bonaventura, C., Bonaventura, J., & Stamler, J. S. (1996): S-nitrosohaemoglobin: a dynamic activity of blood involved in vascular control. *Nature*, 380, 221–226.

Jiang, R., Manson, J. E., Stampfer, M. J., Liu, S., Willet, W. C., & Hu, F. B. (2002): Nut and peanut butter consumption and risk of type 2 diabetes in women. *JAMA*, 288, 2554–2560.

Jones, R. W., Rees, R. W., Minhas, S., Ralph, D., Persad, R. A., & Jeremy, J. Y. (2002): Oxygen free radicals and the penis. *Expert Opinion in Pharmacotherapy*, 3, 889–897.

Juven, B. (1972): Studies on the mechanism of the antimicrobial action of oleuropein. *Journal of Applied Bacteriology*, 35, 559–567.

Kahneman, D., Krueger, A., Schkade, D., Schwarz, N., & Stone, A. (2003): Measuring the quality of experience. Princeton University, working paper.

Kaiser, D. R., Billups, K., Mason, C., Wetterling, R., Lundberg, J. L., & Bank, A. J. (2004): Impaired brachial artery endothelium-dependent and -independent vasodilation in men with erectile dysfunction and no other clinical cardiovascular disease. *Journal of the American College of Cardiology*, 43, 179–184.

Kandeel, F. R., Koussa, V. K. T., & Swerdloff, R. S. (2001): Male sexual function and its disorders: Physiology, pathophysiology, clinical investigation, and treatment. *Endocrine Reviews*, 22, 342-388. Adapted from Swerdloff, R. S., & Kandeel, F. R. (1992): *Textbook of Internal Medicine*. Philadelphia: Lippincott Williams & Wilkins.

Kaneuchi, M., Sasaki, M., Tanka, Y., Yamamoto, R., Sakuragi, N., & Dahiya, R. (2003): Resveratrol suppresses growth of Ishikawa cell through down-regulation of EGF. *International Journal of Oncology*, 23, 1167–1172.

Kang, K., Park, Y., Hwang, H. J., Kim, S. H., Lee, J. G., & Shin, H. C. (2003): Antioxidative properties of brown algae polyphenolics and their perspectives as chemopreventive agents against vascular risk factors. *Archives of Pharmacol Research*, 26, 286–293.

Kaplan, H. S. (1979): *Disorders of Sexual Desire and Other New Concepts and Techniques in Sex Therapy*. New York: Brunner/Mazel Publications.

Kaplan, S. A., Reis, R. B., Kohn, I. J., Ikeguchi, E. F., Laor, E., Te, A. E., & Martins, A. C. (1999): Safety and efficacy of sildenafil in postmenopausal women with sexual dysfunction. *Urology*, 53, 481–486.

Karim, M., McCormick, K., & Kappagoda, C. T. (2000): Effects of cocoa extract on endothelium-dependent relaxation. *Journal of Nutrition*, 30(8 Suppl), S2105–S2108.

Kauhanen, J., Kaplan, G. A., Goldberg, D. E., Salonen, R., & Salonen, J. T. (1999): Pattern of alcohol drinking and progression of atherosclerosis. *Arteriosclerosis, Thrombosis & Vascular Biology*, 19, 3001–3006.

Keevil, J. G., Osman, H. E., Reed, J. D., & Folts, J. D. (2000): Grape juice, but not orange juice or grapefruit juice, inhibits human platelet aggregation. *Journal of Nutrition*, 130, 53–56.

Kelly, G. F. (1994): *Sexuality Today*. Guilford, CT: Dushkin Publishing Group.

Kim, S. W., Paick, J., Park, D. W., Chae, I., & Oh, B. (2001): Potential predictors of asymptomatic ischemic heart disease in patients with vasculogenic erectile dysfunction. *Urology*, 58, 441–445.

Kinsey, A. C., Pomeroy, W. B., & Martin, C. E. (1948): *Sexual behavior in the human male*. Philadelphia, W. B. Saunders Co.

Kinsey, A. C., Pomeroy, W. B., Martin, C. E., & Gebhart, P. H. (1953): *Sexual behavior in the human female*. Philadelphia, W. B. Saunders Co.

Kirby, M., Jackson, G., Betteridge, J., & Friedli, K. (2001): Is erectile dysfunction a marker for cardiovascular disease? *International Journal of Clinical Practice*, 55, 614–618.

Kiss, J. P., Zsilla, G., & Vizi, E. S. (2004): Inhibitory effects on dopamine transporters: interneuronal communication without receptors. *Neurochemistry International*, 45, 485–489.

Klatsky, A. L. (1996): Alcohol, coronary disease, and hypertension. *Annu. Rev. Med*, 47, 149–160. Review.

Klatsky, A. L., Armstrong, M. A., & Friedman, G. D. (1997): Red wine, white wine, liquor, beer, and risk for coronary artery disease hospitalization. *American Journal of Cardiology,* 80, 416–420.

Klatsky, A. L., Friedman, G. D., & Armstrong, M. A. (1986): The relationships between alcoholic beverage use and other traits to blood pressure: a new Kaiser Permanente study. *Circulation,* 73, 628–636.

Kloner, R. A., Mullin, S. H., Shook, T., Matthews, R., Maydella, G., Burstein, S., Peled, H., Pollick, C., Choudhary, R., Rosen, R., & Padma-Nathan, H. (2003): Erectile dysfunction in the cardiac patient: how common and should we treat? *Journal of Urology,* 170, S46–S50.

Knapp, H. R. (1997): Dietary fatty acids in human thrombosis and hemostasis. *American Journal of Clinical Nutrition,* 65, S1687–S1698.

Knopp, R. H., Retzlaff, B., Fish, B., Walden, C., Wallick, S., Anderson, M., Aikawa, K., & Kahn, S. E. (2003): Effects of insulin resistance and obesity on lipoprotein and sensitivity to egg feeding. *Arteriosclerosis, Thrombosis & Vascular Biology,* 23, 1437–1443.

Krauss, R. M. (2001): Atherogenic lipoprotein phenotypes and diet-gene interactions. *Journal of Nutrition,* 131, S340–S343.

Krauss, R. M., & Dreon, D. M. (1995): Low-density-lipoproteins subclasses and response to low-fat diet in healthy men. *American Journal of Clinical Nutrition,* 62, S478–S487.

Kris-Etherton, P. M., Harris, W. S., & Appel, L. J. (2003): Fish consumption, fish oil, omega-3 fatty acids, and cardiovascular disease. *Circulation,* 106, 2747.

Kritchevsky, S. B. (2004): A review of scientific research and recommendations regarding eggs. *Journal of the American College of Nutrition,* 23, S596–S600.

Kritchevsky, S. B., & Kritchevsky, D. (2000): Egg consumption and coronary heart disease: an epidemiological overview. *Journal of the American College of Nutrition,* 19, S549–S555.

Kroll, R. (2004): Testosterone transdermal patches (TTP) significantly improved sexual function in naturally menopausal women in a large phase III study. Presented at the annual meeting of the American Society for Reproductive Medicine, Philadelphia, PA, Oct. 16–20.

Kronmal, R. A., Cain, K. C., Ye, Z., & Omenn, G. S. (1993): Total serum cholesterol levels and mortality risk as a function of age: a report based on the Framingham data. *Archives of Internal Medicine,* 153, 1065–1073.

Lagiou, P., Wuu, J., Trichopoulos, A., Hsieh, C. C., Adami, H. O., & Trichopoulos, D. (1999): Diet and benign prostatic hyperplasia: a study in Greece. *Urology,* 54, 284–290.

Laumann, E. O., Paik, A., & Rosen, R. C. (1999): Sexual dysfunction in the United States: prevalence and predictors. *Journal of the American Medical Association,* 281, 537.

Lee, C. W., & Sheffer, A. L. (2003): Peanut allergy. *Allergy & Asthma Proceedings,* 24, 259–264.

Lee, K. W., Kim, Y. J., & Lee, C. Y. (2003): Cocoa has more phenolic phytochemicals and a higher antioxidant capacity than teas and red wine. *Journal of Agricultural & Food Chemistry,* 51, 7292–7295.

Leighton, F., Cuevas, A., Guash, V., Perez, D. D., Strobel, P., San Martin, A., Urzua, U., Diez, M. S., Foncea, R., Castillo, O., Mizon, C., Espinoza, M. A., Urquiaga, I., Rozowski, J., Maiz, A., & Germain, A. (1999): Plasma polyphenols and antioxidants, oxidative DNA damage and endothelial function in a diet and wine intervention study in humans. *Drugs in Experimental Clinical Research*, 25, 133–141.

Leikert, J. F., Rathel, T. R., Wohlfart, P., Cheynier, V., Vollmar, A. M., & Dirsch, V. M. (2002): Red wine polyphenols enhance endothelial nitric oxide synthase expression and subsequent nitric oxide release from endothelial cells. *Circulation*, 106, 1614–1617.

Levitt, E. E., Konovsky, M., Freese, M. P., & Thompson, J. F. (1979): Intravaginal pressure assessed by Kegel perineometer. *Archives of Sexual Behavior*, 8, 425–430.

Lewis, J. G., Ghanadian, R., & Chisholm, G. D. (1976): Serum 5 alpha-dihydrotestosterone and testosterone changes with age in man. *Acta Endocrinologica* (Copenhagen), 82, 444–448.

Li, X. P., Zhou, Y., Zhao, S. P., Gao, M., Zhou, Q., C., & Li, Y. S. (2004): Effect of endogenous estrogen on endothelial function in women with coronary heart disease and its mechanism. *Clinica Chimica Acta*, 339, 183–188.

Lightner, D. J. (2002): Female sexual dysfunction. *Mayo Clinic Proceedings*, 77, 698–702.

Lind, J. (1753): *A Treatise of the Scurvy*. Edinburgh: A. Kincaid & A. Donaldson.

Linn, S., Carroll, M., Johnson, C., Fulwood, R., Kalsbeek, W., & Briefel, R. (1993): High-density lipoprotein cholesterol and alcohol consumption in US white and black adults. *American Journal of Public Health,* 83 (11 Suppl), 811–816.

Liu, F., Lau, B. H., Peng, Q., & Shah, V. (2000): Pycnogenol protects vascular endothelial cells from beta-amyloid-induced injury. *Biological and Pharmaceutical Bulletin*, 23, 735–737.

Lopez-Garcia, E., & Hu, F. B. (2004): Nutrition and the endothelium. *Current Diabetes Reports*, 4, 253–259.

Mahley, R. W., Palaoglu, K. E., Atak, Z., Dawson-Pepin, J., Langlois, A. M., Cheung, V., Onat, H., Fulks, P., Mahley, L. L., Vakar, F., et al. (1995): Turkish heart study: lipids, lipoproteins, and apolipoproteins. *Journal of Lipid Research*, 36, 839–859.

Marckmann., P., & Gronbaek, M. (1995): Fish consumption and coronary heart disease mortality: a systematic review of prospective cohort studies. *European Journal of Clinical Nutrition*, 53, 585–590.

Marsiglio, W., & Donnelly, D. (1991) Sexual relations in later life: a national study of married persons. *Journal of Gerontology*, 46, S338–S344.

Maskalyk, J. (2002): Grapefruit juice: potential drug interactions. *Canadian Medical Association Journal*, 167, 279–280.

Massaro, M., Carluccio, M. A., & De Caterina, R. (1999): Direct vascular antiatherogenic effects of oleic acid: a clue to the cardioprotective effects of the Mediterranean diet. *Cardiologia*, 44, 507–513.

Masters, W. H., & Johnson, V. E. (1966): *Human Sexual Response*. Boston: Little, Brown & Co.

Masters, W. H., & Johnson, V. E. (1970): *Human Sexual Inadequacy*. Boston: Little, Brown & Co.

Masters, W. H., Johnson, V. E., & Kolodny, R. C. (1997): *Human Sexuality*. New York: Addison-Wesley.

Mathur, S., Devaraj, S., Grundy, S. M., & Jialal, I. (2002): Cocoa products decrease low density lipoprotein oxidative susceptibility but do not affect biomarkers of inflammation in humans. *Journal of Nutrition*, 132, 3663–3667.

Mayor, S. (2004): Pfizer will not apply for a license for sildenafil for women. *British Medical Journal*, 542, 7439–7452.

McCully, K. S. (1969): Vascular pathology of homocysteinemia: implications for the pathogenesis of atherosclerosis. *American Journal of Pathology*, 56, 111–128.

McCully, K. S. (1996): *The Homocysteine Revolution*. New Canaan, CT: Keats.

Mei, Y., Qian, F., Wei, D., & Liu, J. (2004): Reversal of cancer multidrug resistance by green tea polyphenols. *Journal of Pharmacy & Pharmacology*, 56, 1307–1314.

Moncada, S., & Higgs, E. A. (eds.) (1990): *Nitric Oxide from L-arginine: A Bioregulatory System*. Amsterdam: Elsevier Science Publishers.

Moore, B. E., & Rothschild, A. J. (1999): Treatment of antidepressant-induced sexual dysfunction. www.hosppract.com/issues/1999/01/moore.htm.

Moreland, R. B., Goldstein, I., & Traish, A. (1998): Sildenafil, a novel inhibitor of phosphodiesterase type 5 in human corpus cavernosum smooth muscle cells. *Life Sciences*, 62, 309–318.

Morris, M. C., Sacks, F., & Rosner, B. (1993): Does fish oil lower blood pressure? A meta-analysis of controlled trials. *Circulation*, 88, 523–533.

Mosca, L., Grundy, S. M., Judelson, D., King, K., Limacher, M., Oparil, S., Pasternal, R., Pearson, T. A., Redberg, R. F., Smith, S. C., Jr., Winston, M., & Zinberg, S. (1999): AHA/ACC Scientific Statement: Consensus Panel. Guide to preventive cardiology for women. *Journal of the American College of Cardiology*, 33, 1751–1755.

Murabito, J. M., Evans, J. C., Larson, M. G., Nieto, K., Levy, D., & Wilson, P. W. (2003): The Ankle-Brachial Index in the elderly and risk of stroke, coronary disease, and death: the Framingham Study. *Archives of Internal Medicine*, 163, 1939–1942.

Muriana, F. J. (1997): Intake of olive oil can modulate the transbilayer movement of human erythrocyte membrane cholesterol. *Cellular Molecular Life Science*, 53, 469–500.

Naber, K., Ertel, M., Michael, S., Petersohn, C., Bar, P., & Engert, K. (2003): Colleague's tips against recurrent cystitis: cranberry juice instead of antibiotics. *MMW Fortschrift Medizin*, 145, 12–13.

Nawata, H., Kato, K., & Ibayashi, H. (1977): Age-dependent change in serum 5 alpha-dihydrotestosterone and its relation to testosterone in man. *Andocrinologia Japonica*, 24, 41–45.

Ney, P. G. (1986): The intravaginal absorption of male hormones and their possible effect on female behavior. *Medical Hypotheses*, 20, 221–231.

Nikoobakht, M., Nasseh, H., & Pourkasmaee, M. (2005): The relationship between lipid profile and erectile dysfunction. *Int. J. Impot. Res*, 17, 523–526.

No authors listed (date unknown): Female sexual anatomy. Institute for Sexual Medicine, Boston University School of Medicine, Boston, MA.

No authors listed (1998): Healthy Sexuality and Vital Aging. Survey conducted by Roper Starch Worldwide.

No authors listed (2002): Office of Nutritional Products, Labeling, and Dietary Supplements, Center for Food Safety and Applied Nutrition, US Food and Drug Administration. Letter responding to a request to reconsider the qualified claim for a dietary supplement health claim for omega-3 fatty acids and coronary heart disease. Docket No. 91N-0103. February 8, 2002. Available at: www.cfsan.fda.gov/~dms/ds-ltr28.html. Accessed October 3, 2002.

No author listed. (May 2004): What is female sexual dysfunction? Harvard Health Publications—Archived Articles. www.health.harvard.edu/hhp/article/content.do?name=WN0504f.

Node, K., Kitakaze, M., Yoshikawa, H., Kosaka, H., & Hori, M. (1997): Reduced plasma concentrations of nitrogen oxide in individuals with essential hypertension. *Hypertension*, 30, 404–405.

Obisesan, T. O., Hirsch, R., Kosoko, O., Carlson, L., & Parrott, M. (1998): Moderate wine consumption is associated with decreased odds of developing age-related macular degeneration in NHANES-1. *Journal of the American Geriatric Society*, 46, 1–7.

Orshal, J. M., & Khalil, R. A. (2004): Gender, sex hormones, and vascular tone. *American Journal of Physiology. Regulatory, Integrative and Comparative Physiology*, 286, R233–R249.

Pagnotta, P., Germano, G., Filippo, G. G., Rosano, G. M. C., & Chierchia, S. L. (1997): Oral L-arginine supplementation improves essential arterial hypertension. *Circulation*(I Suppl), 96, 3014.

Panagiotakos, D. B., Chrysohoou, C., Pitsavos, C., Skoumas, J., Zeibekis, A., Papaioannou, I., Papadimitriou, L. E., Toutouza, M., Toutouzas, P., & Stefanadis, C. (2003): The prevalence of clinical and biochemical markers related to cardiovascular disease: design and preliminary results from the ATTICA study. *Hellenic Journal of Cardiology*, 44, 308–316.

Park, K., Goldstein, I., Andry, C., Siroky, M. B., Krane, R. J., & Azadzoi, K. M. (1997): Vasculogenic female sexual dysfunction: the hemodynamic basis for vaginal engorgement insufficiency and clitoral erectile insufficiency. *International Journal of Impotence Research*, 9, 27–37.

Park, K., Moreland, R. B., Goldstein, I., Atala, A., Traish, A. (1998): Seldenafil inhibits phosphodiesterase type 5 in human clitoral corpus cavernosum smooth muscle. *Biochemistry & Biophysics Research Communications*, 249, 612–617.

Pearson, T. A. (1996): Alcohol and heart disease (from the Nutrition Committee of the American Heart Association). *Circulation*, 94, 3023–3025.

Perez-Jimenez, F. (1995): Lipoprotein concentrations in normolipidemic males consuming oleic acid-rich diets from two different sources: olive oil and oleic acid-rich sunflower oil. *American Journal of Clinical Nutrition*, 62, 769–775.

Petkov, V. (1978): Pharmacological studies on substances of plant origin with coronary dilatating and antiarrhythmic action. *Comparative Medicine East & West*, 6, 123–130.

Petroni, A. (1995): Inhibition of platelet aggregation and eicosanoid production by phenolic compounds of olive oil. *Thrombosis Research*, 78, 150–151.

Piatti, P. M., Monti, L. D., Valsecchi, G., Magni, F., Setola, E., Marchesi, F., Galli-Kienle, M., Possa, G., & Alberti, K. G. (2001): Long-term oral L-arginine administration improves peripheral and hepatic insulin sensitivity in type 2 diabetic patients. *Diabetes Care*, 24, 875–880.

Picitano, M. C., Curi, R., Machado, U. F., & Carpinelli, A. R. (1998): Soybean- and olive-oil-enriched diets increase insulin secretion to glucose stimulus in isolated pancreatic rat islets. *Physiology & Behavior*, 65, 289–294.

Pignatelli, P., Pulcinelli, F. M., Celestini, A., Lenti, L., Ghiselli, A., Gazzaniga, P. P., & Voli, F. (2000): The flavonoids quercetin and catechin synergistically inhibit platelet function by antagonizing the intracellular production of hydrogen peroxide. *American Journal of Clinical Nutrition*, 72, 1150–1155.

Piletz, J. E., Segraves, K. B., Feng, Y. Z., Maguire, E., Dunger, B., & Halaris, A. (1998): Plasma MHPG response to yohimbine treatment in women with hypoactive sexual desire. *Journal of Sex & Marital Therapy*, 24, 43–54.

Plotnick, G. D., Corretti, M. C., Vogel, R. A., Hesslink, R., Jr., & Wise, J. A. (2003): Effect of supplemental phytonutrients on impairment of the flow-mediated brachial artery vasoactivity after a single high-fat meal. *Journal of the American College of Cardiology*, 41, 1744–1749.

Rajfer, J., Aronson, W. J., Bush, P. A., Dorey, F. J., & Ignarro, L. J. (1992): Nitric oxide as a mediator of relaxation of the corpus cavernosum in response to nonadrenergic, noncholinergic neurotransmission. *New England Journal of Medicine*, 326, 90–94.

Ramirez-Tortosa, M. C., Suarez, A., Gomez, M. C., Mir, A., Ros, E., Mataix, J., & Gil, A. (1999): Effect of extra-virgin olive oil and fish-oil supplementation on plasma lipids and susceptibility of low-density lipoprotein to oxidative alteration in free-living Spanish male patients with peripheral vascular disease. *Clinical Nutrition*, 18, 167–174.

Rayo Llerena, I., & Marin Huerta, E. (1998): Wine and the heart. *Revista Española de Cardiologia*, 51, 435–439.

Rector, T. S., Bank, A. J., Mullen, K. A., Tchumperlin, L. K., Sih, R., Pillai, K., & Kubo, S. H. (1996): Randomized, double-blind, placebo controlled study of supplemental oral L-arginine in patients with heart failure. *Circulation*, 93, 2135–2141.

Renaud, S., & de Lorgeril, M. (1992): Wine, alcohol, platelets, and the French paradox for coronary heart disease. *Lancet*, 20, 1523–1526.

Renaud, S., & Gueguen, R. (1998): The French paradox and wine drinking. *Novartis Foundation Symposium*, 216, 208–217.

Ricci, S., Celani, M. G., Righetti, E., Caruso, A., De Medio, G., Trovarelli, G., Romoli, S., Stragliotto, E., & Spizzichino, L. (1997): Fatty acid dietary intake and the risk of ischaemic stroke: a multicentre case-control study. UFA Study Group. *Journal of Neurology*, 244, 360–364.

Rimm, E. B., Klatsky, A., Grobbee, D., & Stampfer, M. J. (1996): Review of moderate alcohol consumption and reduced risk of coronary heart disease: is the effect due to beer, wine or spirits? *British Medical Journal*, 312, 731–736.

Riquet, A. M., Wolff, N., Laoubi, S., Vergnaud, J. M., & Feigenbaum, A. (1998): Food and packaging interactions: determination of the kinetic parameters of olive oil diffusion in polypropylene using concentration profiles. *Food Additives and Contaminants*, 15, 690–700.

Rizvi, K., Hampson, J. P., & Harvey, J. N. (2002): Do lipid-lowering drugs cause erectile dysfunction? A systematic review. *Family Practice*, 19, 95–98.

Roberts, C. K., Vaziri, N. D., Xiu, Q., Wang, R., & Barnard, R. J. (2000): Enhanced

NO inactivation and hypertension induced by a high-fat, refined-carbohydrate diet. *Hypertension*, 36, 423–429.

Roberts, K., Dunn, K., Jean, S. K., & Lardinois, C. K. (2000): Syndrome X: medical nutrition therapy. *Nutritional Review*, 58, 154–160, review.

Rosen, R. C., Riley, A., Wagner, G., Osterloh, I. H., Kirkpatrick, J., & Mishra, A. (1997): The International Index of Erectile Function (IIEF): a multidimensional scale for assessment of erectile dysfunction. *Urology*, 49, 822–830.

Roumegerre, T., Wespes, E., Carpentier, Y., Hoffmann, P., & Schulmann, C. C. (2003): Erectile dysfunction is associated with a high prevalence of hyperlipidemia and coronary heart disease risk. *European Urology*, 44, 355–359.

Ruiz-Gutierrez, V. (1996): Plasma lipids, erythrocyte membrane lipids and blood pressure of hypertensive women after ingestion of dietary oleic acid from two different sources. *Journal of Hypertension*, 14, 1483–1490.

Ruiz-Gutierrez, V., Perona, J. S., Pacheco, Y. M., Muriana, F. J., & Villar, J. (1999): Incorporation of dietary triacylglycerols from olive oil and high-oleic sunflower oil into VLDL triacylglycerols of hypertensive patients. *European Journal of Clinical Nutrition*, 53, 687–693.

Rush, C. (2003): Finally, how to find and love your G-spot. *Cosmopolitan*, 235, 210–213.

Sacco, R. L., Elkind, M., Boden-Albala, B., Lin, I. F., Kargman, D. E., Hauser, W. A., Shea, S., & Paik, M. C. (1999): The protective effects of moderate alcohol consumption on ischemic stroke. *Journal of the American Medical Association*, 281, 53–60.

Sah, J. F., Balasubramanian, S., Eckert, R. L., & Rorke, E. A. (2004): Epigallocatechin-3-gallate inhibits epidermal growth factor receptor signaling pathway. Evidence for direct inhibition of ERK1/2 and AKT kinases. *J. Biol. Chem.*, 9, 12755–12762. Epub Dec 29, 2003.

Salonen, J. T, Seppanen, K., Lakka, T. A., Salonen, R., & Kaplan, G. A. (2000): Mercury accumulation and accelerated progression of carotid atherosclerosis: a population-based prospective 4-year follow-up study in men in eastern Finland. *Atherosclerosis*, 148: 265–273.

Salonia, A., Munarriz, R., & Montorsi, F. (2004): Vascular aetiology of female sexual arousal disorder (FSAD) in women (sic): evidence and diagnostic approach. *Urodinamica*, 14, 94–98.

Saltzman, E. A., Guay, A. T., & Jacobson, J. (2004): Improvement in erectile function in men with organic erectile dysfunction by correction of elevated cholesterol levels: a clinical observation. *Journal of Urology*, 172, 255–258.

Sauvaget, C., Nagano, J., Allen, N., & Kodama, K. (2003): Vegetable and fruit intake and stroke mortality in the Hiroshima/Nagasaki Life Span Study. *Stroke*, 34, 2355–2360.

Schachter, M. (2000): Erectile dysfunction and lipid disorders. *Current Medical Research Opinion*, 16, 1:S9–12.

Schiavi, R. C., Schreiner-Engel, P., Mandeli, J., Schanzer H., & Cohen E. (1990): Healthy aging and male sexual function. *Am. J. Psychiatry*, 147, 766–771.

Schwitters, B., & Masquelier, J. (1993): *OPC in Practice*. Rome: Alpha Omega Editrice.

Sharma, G., Tyagi, A. K., Singh, R. P., Chan, D. C., & Agarwal, R. (2004): Synergistic anti-cancer effects of grape seed extract and conventional cytotoxic agent doxorubicin against human breast carcinoma cells. *Breast Cancer Research & Treatment*, 85, 1–12.

Shiri, R., Koskimaki, J., Hakam, M., Hakkinen, J., Tammela, T. L., Huhtala, B., & Auvinen, A. (2003): Effect of chronic diseases on incidence of erectile dysfunction. *Urology*, 62, 1097–1102.

Sierksma, A., van der Gaag, M. S., Grobbee, D. E., & Hendriks, H. F. (2003): Acute and chronic effects of dinner with alcoholic beverages on nitric oxide metabolites in healthy men. *Clinical & Experimental Pharmacology and Physiology*, 30, 504–506.

Sies, H., & Stahl, W. (2004): Carotenoids and UV protection. *Photochemical & Photobiological Sciences*, 3, 749–752.

Simonsen, U., Garcia-Sacristan, A., & Prieto, D. (2002): Penile arteries and erection. *Journal of Vascular Research*, 39, 283–303.

Singh, R. P., Tyagi, A. K., Dhanalakshmi, S., Agarwal, R., Agarwal, C. (2004): Grape seed extract inhibits advanced human prostate tumor growth and angiogenesis and upregulates insulin-like growth factor binding protein 3. *International Journal of Cancer*, 108, 733–740.

Siroky, M. B., & Azadzoi, K. M. (2003): Vasculogenic erectile dysfunction: newer therapeutic strategies. *Journal of Urology*, 170, S24–S29; discussion S29–S30.

Slob, A. K., Buitenhuis, E. F., Gijs, L., & Hop, W. C. (2001): Leiden Impotence Screening Test (LIST) in men with erectile dysfunction as a pre-selective method prior to psychophysiological diagnostic tests. *Nederlands Tijsschrift Geneeskunde*, 145, 581–586.

Sodeman, W. A., & Sodeman, T. M. (1979): *Pathological Physiology*. 6th ed. Philadelphia: W. B. Saunders.

Solomon, H., Man, J. W., & Jackson, G. (2003): Erectile dysfunction and the cardiovascular patient: endothelial dysfunction is the common denominator. *Heart*, 89, 251–253.

Sommerburg, O., Keunen, J. E., Bird, A. C., & van Kujik, F. J. (1998): Fruits and vegetables that are sources for lutein and zeaxanthin: the macular pigment in human eyes. *British Journal of Ophthalmology*, 82, 907–910.

Speckens, A. E., Hengeveld, M. W., Lycklama, A., Nijeholt, G. A., van Hemert, A. M., & Hawton, K. E. (1993): Discrimination between psychogenic and organic erectile dysfunction. *Journal of Psychosomatic Medicine*, 37, 135–145.

Speel, T. G., van Langen, H., & Meuleman, E. J. (2003): The risk of coronary heart disease in men with erectile dysfunction. *European Journal of Urology*, 44, 366–370.

Srilatha, B., Adaikan, P. G., Ng, S. C., & Arulkumara, S. (1999): Elevated low-density lipoprotein cholesterol (LDL-C) enhances pro-erectile neurotransmission in the corpus cavernosum. *International Journal of Impotence Research*, 11, 159–165.

Stamler, J., Daviglus, M. L., Garside, D. B., Dyer, A. R., Greenland, P., & Neaton, J. D. (2002): Relationship of baseline serum cholesterol levels in 3 large cohorts of younger men to long-term coronary, cardiovascular, and all-cause mortality and longevity. *Journal of the American Medical Association,* 284, 311–318.

Stamler, J. S., Loh, E., Roddy, M-A., Currie, K. E., & Creager, M. A. (1994): Nitric oxide regulates basal systemic and pulmonary vascular resistance in healthy humans. *Circulation*, 89, 2035–2040.

Stanislavov, R., & Nikolova, V. (2003): Treatment of erectile dysfunction with pycnogenol and L-arginine. *Journal of Sex and Marital Therapy*, 29, 207–213.

Starr, B. D., & Weiner, M. B. (1982): *The Starr-Weiner Report on Sex and Sexuality in the Mature Years*. New York: McGraw-Hill.

Stenn, K. S., & Paus, R. (2001): Controls of hair follicle cycling. *Physiological Reviews*, 81, 449–494.

Stoclet, J. C., Kleschyov, A., Andriambeloson, E., Diebolt, M., & Andriantsito-haina, R. (1999): Endothelial NO release caused by red wine polyphenols. *Journal of Physiology & Pharmacology*, 50, 535–540.

Stone, N. J. (1996): Fish consumption, fish oil, lipids, and coronary heart disease. *Circulation*, 94, 2337–2340.

Sullivan, M. E., Keoghane, S. R., & Miller, M. A. (2001): Vascular risk factors and erectile dysfunction. *British Journal of Urology*, 87, 838–845.

Sullivan, M. E., Miller, M. A., Bell, C. R., Jagroop, I. A., Thompson, C. S., Khna, M. A., Morgan, R. J., & Mikhailidis, D. P. (2001): Fibrinogen, lipoprotein (a) and lipids in patients with erectile dysfunction: a preliminary study. *International Angiology*, 20, 195–199.

Sun, J., Chu, Y. F., Wu, X., & Liu, R. H. (2002): Antioxidant and antiproliferative activities of common fruits. *Journal of Agricultural Food Chemistry*, 50, 7449–7454.

Surdacki, A., Nowicki, M., Sandmann, J., Tsikas, D., Boeger, R. H., Bode-Boeger, S. M., Kruszelnicka-Kwiatkowska, O., Kokot, F., Dubiel, J. S., & Froelich, J. C. (1999): Reduced urinary excretion of nitric oxide metabolites and increased plasma levels of asymmetrical dimethylarginine in men with essential hypertension. *Journal of Cardiovascular Pharmacology*, 33, 652–658.

Taguri, T., Tanaka, T., & Kouno, I. (2004): Antimicrobial activity of 10 different plant polyphenols against bacteria causing food-borne disease. *Biological Pharmacology Bulletin*, 27, 1965–1969.

Takahashi, T., Kamyia, T., Hasegawa, A., & Yokoo, Y. (1999): Procyanidin oligomers selectively and intensively promote proliferation of mouse hair epithelial cells in vitro and active hair follicle growth in vivo. *Journal of Investigative Dermatology*, 112, 310–316.

Takahashi, T., Kamiya, T., & Yokoo, Y. (1998): Proanthocyanidins from grape seeds promote proliferation of mouse hair follicle cells in vitro and convert hair cycle in vivo. *Acta Dermato-Venereologica*, 78, 428–432.

Takahashi, T., Yokoo, Y., Inoue, T., & Ishii, A. (1999): Toxicological studies on procyanidin B-2 for external application as a hair growing agent. *Food & Chemical Toxicology*, 37, 545–552.

Talley, J. D., & Crawley, I. S. (1985): Transdermal nitrate, penile erection, and spousal headache. *Annals of Internal Medicine*, 103, 804.

Tassou, C. (1995): Inhibition of *Salmonella enteritidis* by oleuropein in broth and in a model food system. *Letters in Applied Microbiology*, 20, 120–124.

Tavris, C., & Sadd, S. (1977): *The Redbook Report on Female Sexuality*. New York: Delacorte.

Thun, M. J., Peto, R., Lopez, A. D., Monaco, J. H., Henley, S. J., Heath, C. W., Jr., & Doll, E. (1997): Alcohol consumption and mortality among middle-aged and elderly US adults. *New England Journal of Medicine,* 337, 1705–1714.

Tjonneland, A., Gronbaek, M., Stripp, C., & Overvad, K. (1999): Wine intake and diet in a random sample of 48,763 Danish men and women. *American Journal of Clinical Nutrition,* 69, 49–54.

Toesca, A., Stolfi, V.M., & Cocchia, D. (1996): Immunohistochemical study of the corpora cavernosa of the human clitoris. *J. Anat*, 188 (PL 3), 513–520.

Tortora, G. J., & Anagnostakos, N. P. (1984): *Principles of Anatomy and Physiology*. 4th ed. New York: Harper & Row.

Tranter, H. S. (1993): The effect of the olive phenolic compound, oleuprotein, on growth and enterotoxin B production by *Staphylococcus aureus*. *Journal of Applied Bacteriology*, 74, 253–259.

Trichopoulou, A., & Critselis, E. (2004): Mediterranean diet and longevity. *European Journal of Cancer Prevention*, 13, 453–456.

Trichopoulou, A., & Vasilopoulou, E. (2000): Mediterranean diet and longevity. *British Journal of Nutrition*, 84(2 Suppl): S205–S209.

Tsimikas, S., Philis-Tsimikas, A., Alexopoulos, S., Sigari, F., Lee, C., & Reaven, P. D. (1999): LDL isolated from Greek subjects on a typical diet or from American subjects on an oleate-supplemented diet induces less monocyte chemotaxis and adhesion when exposed to oxidative stress. *Arteriosclerosis, Thrombosis & Vascular Biology*, 19, 122–130.

Tucker, K. L. (2004): Dietary intake and coronary heart disease: A variety of nutrients and phytochemicals are [sic] important. *Current Treatment Options in Cardiovascular Medicine*, 6, 291–302.

Tunstall-Pedoe, H., Kuulasmaa, K., Mahonen, M., Tolonen, H., Ruokokoski, E., & Amouyel, P. (1999): Contribution of trends in survival and coronary-event rates to changes in coronary heart disease mortality: 10-year results from 37 WHO MONICA project populations: monitoring trends and determinants in cardiovascular disease. *Lancet*, 353, 1547–1557.

Tzonou, A., Signorello, L. B., Lagiou, P., Wuu, J., Trichopoulos, D., & Trichopoulos, A. (1999): Diet and cancer of the prostate: a case-control study in Greece. *International Journal of Cancer*, 80, 704–708.

Uchida, S., Ikari, N., Ohta, H., Niwa, M., Nonaka, G., Nishioka, I., & Ozaki, M. (1987): Inhibitory effects of condensed tannins on angiotensin converting enzyme. *Japan Journal of Pharmacology*, 43, 242–246.

Umar, A., Guerin, V., Renard, M., Boisseau, M., Garreau, C., Begaud, B., Molimar, M., & Moore, N. (2003): Effects of Armagnac extracts on human platelet function in vitro and on rat arteriovenous shunt thrombosis in vivo. *Thrombosis Research*, 110, 135–140.

US Environmental Protection Agency. Fish Advisories web page. Available at: www.epa.gov/waterscience/fish/. Accessed October 3, 2002.

US Food and Drug Administration, Center for Food Safety and Applied Nutrition, Office of Seafood. Mercury Levels in Seafood Species. May 2001. Available at: www.cfsan.fda.gov/~frf/sea-mehg.html. Accessed October 3, 2002.

van den Hoogen, P. C. W., Feskens, E. J. M., Nagelkerke, N. J. D., Menotti, A., Nissinen, A., & Kromhout, D. (2000): The relation between blood pressure and mortality due to coronary heart disease among men in different parts of the world. *New England Journal of Medicine*, 342, 1–7.

Verhagen, H., Poulsen, H. E., Loft, S., van Poppel, G., Willems, M. I., & Bladeren, P. J. (1995): Reduction of oxidative DNA-damage in humans by brussels sprouts. *Carcinogenesis*, 16, 969–970.

Visek, W. J. (1986): Arginine needs, physiological state and usual diets: a reevaluation. *Journal of Nutrition*, 116, 36–46.

Visioli, F. (1994): Oleuropein protects low density lipoproteins from oxidation. *Life Science*, 55, 1965–1971.

Visioli, F. (1995): Low density lipoprotein oxidation is inhibited in vitro by olive oil constituents. *Atherosclerosis*, 117, 25–32.

Visioli, F. (1998): Free radical-scavenging properties of olive oil polyphenols. *Biochemical & Biophysical Research Communications*, 247, 60–64.

Visioli, F., Bellosta, S., & Galli, C. (1998): Oleuropein, the bitter principle of olives, enhances nitric oxide production by mouse macrophages. *Life Sciences*, 62, 541–546.

Voght, H. J., Brandl, P., Kockott, G., Schmitz, J. R., Wiegand, M. H., Shadrack, J., & Gierend, M. (1997): Double-blind, placebo-controlled safety and efficacy trial with yohimbine hydrochloride in the treatment of nonorganic erectile dysfunction. *International Journal of Impotence Research*, 9, 155–161.

Vognild, E., Elvevoll, E. O., Brox, J., Olsen, R. L., Barstad, H., Aursand, M., & Osterud, B. (1998): Effects of dietary marine oils and olive oil on fatty acid composition, platelet membrane fluidity, platelet responses, and serum lipids in healthy humans. *Lipids*, 33, 427–436.

Wagner, A. K. (no date given): Selective serotonin reuptake inhibitors and sexual dysfunction: a historical review of the development of evidence for an adverse effect. www.hsph.harvard.edu/Organizations/DDIL/SSRI.htm.

Wagner, G., & Green, R. (1981): *Impotence: Physiological, Psychological, Surgical Diagnosis and Treatment*. New York: Plenum Press.

Wakatsuki, A., Ikenoue, N., Shinohara, K., Watanabe, K., & Fukaya, T. (2004): Small low-density lipoprotein particles and endothelium-dependent vasodilation in postmenopausal women. *Atherosclerosis*, 177, 329–336.

Walczak, M. K., Lokhandwala, N., Hodge, M. B., & Guay, A. T. (2002): Prevalence of cardiovascular risk factors in erectile dysfunction. *Journal of Gender Specific Medicine*, 5, 19–24.

Wallerath, T., Deckert, G., Ternes, T., Anderson, H., Li, H., Witte, K., & Fortermann, U. (2002): Resveratrol, a polyphenolic phytoalexin present in red wine, enhances expression and activity of endothelial nitric oxide synthase. *Circulation*, 106, 1652–1658.

Walton, B., & Thorton, T. (2003): Female sexual dysfunction. *Current Women's Health Reports*, 3, 319–326.

Wang, H., Cao, G., & Prior, R. L. (1996): Total antioxidant capacity of fruits. *Journal of Agriculture & Food Chemistry*, 44, 701–705.

Wang, J., Brown, M. A., Tam, S. H., Chan, M. C., & Whitworth, J. A. (1997): Effects of diet on measurement of nitric oxide metabolites. *Clinical and Experimental Pharmacology & Physiology*, 24, 418–420.

Wang, J. F., Schramm, D. D., Holt, R. R., Ensunsa, J. L., Fraga, C. G., Schmitz, H. H., & Keen, C. L. (2000): A dose-response effect from chocolate consumption on plasma epicatechin and oxidative damage. *Journal of Nutrition*, 130(8 Suppl), S2115–S2119.

Warner, J., & Nazario, B. (1997): Why women lose interest in sex. http://my.webmd.com/content/article/83/97902.htm?z=2953_00000_5023_pe_02.

Watemberg, N., Urkin, Y., & Witztum, A. (1991): Phytophotodermatitis. *Cutis: Cutaneous Medicine for the Practitioner*, 48, 151–152.

Way, T. D., Lee, H. H., Kao, M. C., & Lin, J. K. (2004): Black tea polyphenols theaflavins inhibit aromatase activity and attenuate tamoxifen resistance in HER2/neu-transfected human breast cancer cells through tyrosine kinase suppression. *European Journal of Cancer*, 40, 2164–2174.

Webster, R. (1996): *Why Freud Was Wrong: Sin, Science and Psychoanalysis*. New York: Basic Books.

Wei, M., Macera, C. A., Davis, D. R., Hornung, C. A., Nankin, H. R., & Blair, S. N. (1994): Total cholesterol and high density lipoprotein cholesterol as important predictors of erectile dysfunction. *American Journal of Epidemiology*, 140, 930–937.

Wennmalam, A., Benthin, G., Edlund, A., Jungersten, L., Kieler-Jensen, N., Lundin, S., Nathorst, U., Peterson, A.-S., & Waagstein, F. (1993): Metabolism and excretion of nitric oxide in humans. *Circulation Research*, 73, 1121–1127.

Whipple, B. (2002): Women's sexual pleasure and satisfaction: a new view of female sexual function. *The Female Patient*, 27, 39–44.

Whipple, B., & Brash-McGreer, K. (1997): Management of female sexual dysfunction. In Sipski, M. L., & Alexander, C. J., eds. *Sexual Function in People with Disability and Chronic Illness: A Health Professional's Guide*. Gaithersburg, MD: Aspen Publishers, 509–534.

Willett, W. C. (2001): *Eat, Drink and Be Healthy: The Harvard Medical School Guide to Healthy Eating*. New York: Simon & Schuster Source.

Wincze, J. P., & Carey, M. P. (1991): *Sexual Function*. New York: Guilford Press.

Witteman, J. C., Willett, W. C., Stampfer, M. J., Colditz, G. A., Kok, F. J., Sacks, F. M., Speizer, F. E., Rosner, B., & Hennekens, C. H. (1990): Relation of moderate alcohol consumption and risk of systemic hypertension in women. *American Journal of Cardiology*, 65, 633–637.

Working Group on a New View of Women's Sexual Problems (2000): A new view of women's sexual problems. *Electronic Journal of Human Sexuality*, 3, www.ejhs.org/volume 3/newview.htm. Accessed March 21, 2005.

Wu, A. H., Tseng, C. C., van den Berg, D., & Yu, M. C. (2003): Tea intake, COMT genotype, and breast cancer in Asian-American women. *Cancer Research*, 63, 7526–7529.

Yeatman, T. J., Risley, G. L., & Brunson, M. E. (1991): Depletion of dietary arginine inhibits growth of metastatic tumor. *Arch. Surg*, 126, 1376–1381; discussion 1381–1382.

Zambon, A., Sartore, G., Passera, D., Francini-Pesenti, F., Bassi, A., Basso, C., Zambon, S., Manzato, E., & Crepaldi, G. (1999): Effects of hypocaloric dietary treatment enriched in oleic acid on LDL and HDL subclass distribution in mildly obese women. *Journal of Internal Medicine*, 246, 191–201.

Zarzuelo, A. (1991): Vasodilator effect of olive leaf. *Planta Medica*, 57, 417–419.

Zeisel, S. H., Mar, M.-H., Howe, J. C., & Holden, J. M. (2003): Concentrations of choline-containing compounds and betaine in common foods. *Journal of Nutrition*, 133, 1302–1307.

Zhao, J., Wang, J., Chen, Y., & Agarwal, R. (1999): Anti-tumor-promoting activity of a polyphenolic fraction isolated from grape seeds in the mouse skin two-stage initiation-promotion protocol and identification of procyanidin B5-3'-gallate as the most effective antioxidant constituent. *Carcinogenesis*, 20, 1737–1745.

Zorgniotti, A. W., & Lizza, E. F. (1994): Effect of large doses of nitric oxide precursor, L-arginine, on erectile dysfunction. *International Journal of Impotence Research*, 6, 33–36.

Websites

www.ars.usda.gov/is/AR/archives/nov97/musc1197.htm

www.athealth.com/Practitioner/ceduc/physalguide.html

www.bumc.bu.edu/Dept/Content.aspx?DepartmentID=371&PageID=7305

www.burgundy-talent.com/compnew/english/health/resveratrol.htm

www.cfsan.fda.gov/~frf/sea-mehg.html

www.clinicaltrials.gov/ct/gui/show/NCT00069654

www.datamonitor.com/~2bbf82da36b94b5aa3c760fbee2ea5e0~/all/news/product.asp
    ?pid=0033901A-F384-4A0B-A5A9-AF0D14901DF1

www.earthy.com/goto.htm

www.english.pravda.ru/fun/2002/04/02/27302.html

www.epa.gov/waterscience/fish

www.ers.usda.gov/publications/foodreview/dec2002/

www.fas.usda.gov/info/agexporter/1999/articles/urban.html

www.fjkluth.com/daily.html

www.heartinfo.org/ms/news/523552/main.html

www.herpes.com/nutrition.shtml

http://hunterdonhealthcare.org/WebMD/ConditionsM<ens_Anatomy_Penis.asp

www.mcauley.acu.edu.au/~yuri/aged/Elder1.htm

www.nalusda.gov/fnic/foodcomp/

www.ncbi.nlm.nih.gov.80/entrez/query.fcgi?CMD=Text&DB=PubMed

www.news.cornell.edu/Chronicle/98/2.5.98/resveratrol.htm

www.nutritiondata.com/

www.people.virginia.edu/~rjh9u/impotent.html

www.renewalsresearch.com

www.sexualhealth.com/article.php?Action=read&article_id=401

www.soupsong.com/folives.html

www.theolivepress.com

www.wholehealthmd.com

Index

Page numbers in *italics* refer to illustrations.

hypoactive sexual desire (*cont'd.*)
    nonpharmacological therapy for,
        31–32
    sexual pharmacology for, 32–33

Ignarro, L. J., xxii
immune system, 75
impotence. *See* erectile dysfunction (ED)
indole carbinol 3, 117
infection, 233
insulin, 158
intimacy, 21
    aging and, 21
Italian Vegetable Bake, 210

Japan, 55, 56
Jerusalem artichoke, 68–69
Johnson, Samuel, 28
*Journal of Cardiovascular
    Pharmacology,* 59
Journal of Sex and Medical Therapy,
    77
juices, fruit, 131–32

kale, 69
Kebabs, Scallop, 202
Kegel, Dr. Arnold, 31
Kegel exercises, 31–32
kidney beans, 65
kidneys, 46, 49, 109
Kinsey, A. C., 23, 228–29
    *Sexual Behavior in the Human
        Female,* 229
    Sexual Behavior in the Human Male,
        229
kiwi fruit, 127–28

labia majora, 10, *10*
labia minora, 10, *10,* 17, 24
lamb, 99–100
    foreshank, 99
    ground, 99
    leg, 99
    rib, 100
La Rochefoucauld, 167
Lasagne, Zucchini, 209–10
LDL cholesterol, 6, 44–45, 52–54, 55,
    57, 59, 60, 75, 76–77, 105, 106
lecithin, 86
leeks, 120

legumes, 39, 47, 60
    Greens and Beans, 58–73
    See also beans
Leiden Impotence questionnaire (LIQ),
    33–35
lemon, 108
    Tropical Shrimp Salad, 177
    Very Lemony Chicken, 200
lettuce, 69
Levitra, xxiii, 13, 38
libido, xxiii, 13, 18
    low, in men, 35, 38, 40, 231
    low, in women, xxiii, xxiv, 13, 22, 27,
        28–33, 38, 54, 231
    See also desire
lignans, 118
lima beans, 64
Limas and Spinach, 212
Lind, Dr. James, 76, 116
lithium, 19, 30
lobster, 96
Los Angeles Times, 113
lubricants, 12, 22, 232–33
    application of, 12
    types of, 233
lubrication, vaginal. *See* vaginal
    lubrication
lunch, 155, 165
lungs, 46, 109
lutein, 86, 117–18
lycopene, 115, 117, 122–23
    sources of, 117
lymphocytes, 75
lysine, 77, 82

macadamia nuts, 84
Macaroni and Bean Soup, 189–90
mackerel, 91
macrophages, 53, 54, 75, 77, 106
macular degeneration, 106, 146
mad cow disease, 97
mahimahi, 94
male pattern baldness, 36, 37, 147
male sexual dysfunction, xx, xxii, 3,
    14–23, 33–42
    causes classified by clinical
        manifestations, 40–41
    desire disorders, 35, 38, 40
    ejaculation disorders, 19, 22, 35,
        40–41

platelet aggregation, 51–52, 134, 139
plums, 130
Poached Pears, Maple, 225
pollack, 94
polyphenols, 114–18, 134
    ORAC value of, 112
pomegranate, 130
pomegranate juice, 132
pork, 100
    leg, 100
    sirloin, 100
postmenopausal women, 17, 23, 28, 29, 57
potatoes, 59, 70–71, 108
    Garlic Mashed Potatoes, 214
    sweet, 122
poultry, 39, 80, 100–103
    chicken and cornish hens, 101
    duck, 101
    entrées, 197–5
    game, 103
    goose, 101
    turkey, 101–2
    See also specific poultry
pregnancy, 90
premature ejaculation (PE), 35, 40–41
prescription medications, 9, 17–20
    sexual dysfunction caused by, 17–20, 29–30, 40, 41
    side effects of, 15, 17–20, 29–30, 40, 41
    See also specific medications
prescription sex drugs, xix, xxiii, 9, 13, 16, 22, 38, 47, 48, 49, 50, 231
    development of, xxiii
    risks of, xxiii
    for women, 13, 17, 32
    See also specific drugs
priapism, 41
proanthocyanidins, 118, 145–46
Proctor & Gamble Pharmaceuticals, 32
Profile of Female Sexual Function (PFSF), 32, 33
Propecia, 37
prostate, 7, 8–9, 11
    cancer, 36, 115, 132, 145
    enlargement, 23, 36, 115

protein, 62, 78
    average per capita intake of, 80–81
    in Brights, 118–32
    in Greens and Beans, 62–73
    in Staminators, 74–103
Prozac, 19, 20, 30
prune juice, 132
Pumpkin Pie, Crunchy, 222–23
pycnogenol, 77, 116–17

quercetin, 118
Quesadillas, Guiltless, 193–94

radiation, 105, 106
radishes, 121
Rainbow Honey-Glazed Fruit Salad, 217
Raisin-Carrot Bread, 220
rapid ejaculation (RE), 35
raspberries, 130–31
Ratatouille, Chicken, 198
recipes, 167–227
red beans, 64
    New Orleans Red Beans, 207
Red-Hot Fusilli, 213
red wine, 134–35, 136, 138–39, 145, 161
refined sugars, 44, 157–58
Renaud, Serge, 135
"Report of the International Consensus Development Conference on Female Sexual Dysfunction: Definitions and Classifications," 23–24
reserpine, 19, 30
resveratrol, 118, 127
    in wine, 136–39
rice:
    Black Beans with, 206
    Oriental, 215
    Sunshine, 216
Rockport Fish Chowder, 191–92
romance, 234
RWPCs, 134–35

SAD, 142, 154, 157
salads, 175–87, 221
    Creamy Yogurt Dressing, 184
    Curtido Cabbage Salvadore, 175
    Easy Vinaigrette Salad Dressing, 183
    Fresh Cabbage and Tomato, 178

ABOUT THE AUTHORS

ROBERT FRIED, PH.D., is senior professor of biopsychology at Hunter College, City University of New York. He is a member of the American Physiology Society (APS) (cardiovascular and respiration divisions) and the American Psychological Association (APA). A fellow of the New York Academy of Sciences, Dr. Fried lectures in the US and abroad on cardiovascular function. He has appeared on national and international TV, including CNN and Fox News. He is the author of *The Arginine Solution: The First Guide to America's New Cardio-Enhancing Supplement* and *Breathe Well, Be Well: A Program to Relieve Stress, Anxiety, Asthma, Hypertension, Migraine, and Other Disorders for Better Health*. Dr. Fried lives in New York City.

LYNN EDLEN-NEZIN, PH.D., is director of behavioral science and vice president of strategic planning and research for Grey Healthcare Group. She is a graduate of the doctoral program in clinical health psychology at the Albert Einstein College of Medicine, and completed her internship at the Obesity Research Center at St. Luke's–Roosevelt Hospital Center. She is an American College of Sports Medicine certified personal trainer. Dr. Edlen-Nezin has contributed to several books, and her articles have appeared in magazines including *Self* and *Seventeen,* as well as in the New York *Daily News*. She lives in Jackson Heights, Queens.

ABOUT THE TYPE

This book was set in Sabon, a typeface designed by the well-known German typographer Jan Tschichold (1902–74). Sabon's design is based upon the original letter forms of Claude Garamond and was created specifically to be used for three sources: foundry type for hand composition, Linotype, and Monotype. Tschichold named his typeface for the famous Frankfurt typefounder Jacques Sabon, who died in 1580.